Guidelines for the Psychosocially Assisted Pharmacological Treatment of Opioid Dependence

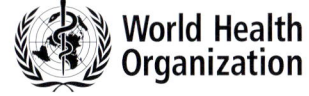

WHO Library Cataloguing-in-Publication Data

Guidelines for the psychosocially assisted pharmacological treatment of opioid dependence.

1.Opioid-related disorders - drug therapy. 2.Opioid-related disorders - psychology. 3.Substance abuse - prevention and control. 4.Guidelines. I.World Health Organization. Dept. of Mental Health and Substance Abuse.

ISBN 978 92 4 154754 3   (NLM classification: WM 284)

© World Health Organization 2009

All rights reserved. Publications of the World Health Organization can be obtained from WHO Press, World Health Organization, 20 Avenue Appia, 1211 Geneva 27, Switzerland (tel.: +41 22 791 3264; fax: +41 22 791 4857; e-mail: bookorders@who.int). Requests for permission to reproduce or translate WHO publications – whether for sale or for noncommercial distribution – should be addressed to WHO Press, at the above address (fax: +41 22 791 4806; e-mail: permissions@who.int).

The designations employed and the presentation of the material in this publication do not imply the expression of any opinion whatsoever on the part of the World Health Organization concerning the legal status of any country, territory, city or area or of its authorities, or concerning the delimitation of its frontiers or boundaries. Dotted lines on maps represent approximate border lines for which there may not yet be full agreement.

The mention of specific companies or of certain manufacturers' products does not imply that they are endorsed or recommended by the World Health Organization in preference to others of a similar nature that are not mentioned. Errors and omissions excepted, the names of proprietary products are distinguished by initial capital letters.

All reasonable precautions have been taken by the World Health Organization to verify the information contained in this publication. However, the published material is being distributed without warranty of any kind, either expressed or implied. The responsibility for the interpretation and use of the material lies with the reader. In no event shall the World Health Organization be liable for damages arising from its use.

Book design by Zando Escultura

Printed in Spain

Contents

Acknowledgements..iv

Abbreviations and acronyms...ix

Executive summary..x
Summary of recommendations..xiv

1 Scope and purpose...1

2 Method of formulating recommendations...3
2.1 Conventions for reporting clinical trial data...4

3 Background..5
3.1 Opioid dependence...5
3.2 Neurobiological aspects of opioid dependence..5
3.3 Epidemiology of illicit opioid use and dependence...6
3.4 Harms associated with opioid use..6
3.5 Economic consequences of opioid use...6
3.6 Natural history of opioid dependence..6
3.7 Opioid dependence as a medical condition...6
3.8 Treatment of opioid dependence...7
   3.8.1 Management of opioid withdrawal..7
   3.8.2 Agonist maintenance treatment..7
   3.8.4 Psychosocial assistance..7

4 Guidelines for health systems at national and subnational levels...............................8
4.1 International regulations..8
4.2 Opioid dependence as a health-care issue..8
4.3 National treatment policy..8
4.4 Ethical issues..9
   4.4.1 Compulsory and coerced treatment..9
   4.4.2 Central registration of patients..10
4.5 Funding..10
4.6 Coverage..11
   4.6.1 Primary care...11
   4.6.2 Prisons..12
4.7 What treatments should be available?..12
4.8 Supervision of dosing for methadone and buprenorphine maintenance............................13

5 Programme level guidelines – for programme managers and clinical leaders.........14
5.1 Clinical governance..14
5.2 Ethical principles and consent..14
5.3 Staff and training..15
   5.3.1 Medical staff...15
   5.3.2 Pharmacy staff...15
   5.3.3 Psychosocial support staff..16
5.4 Clinical records...16

5.5	Medication safety	16
5.6	Treatment provision	17
	5.6.1 Clinical guidelines	17
	5.6.2 Treatment policies	17
	5.6.3 Involuntary discharge and other forms of limit setting	17
	5.6.4 Individual treatment plans	18
	5.6.5 Range of services to be provided	19
	5.6.6 Treatment of comorbid conditions	19
	5.6.7 Psychosocial and psychiatric support	19
	5.6.8 TB, hepatitis and HIV	20
	5.6.9 Hepatitis B vaccination	21
5.7	Treatment evaluation	21
6	**Patient level guidelines – for clinicians**	**23**
6.1	Diagnosis and assessment of opioid dependence	23
	6.1.1 urine drug screening	24
	6.1.2 Testing for infectious diseases	24
	6.1.3 Identifying the patient	24
	6.1.4 Completing the assessment	24
	6.1.4 Diagnostic criteria	25
	6.1.5 Making the diagnosis	25
6.2	Choice of treatment approach	26
6.3	Opioid agonist maintenance treatment	29
	6.3.1 Indications for opioid agonist maintenance treatment	29
	6.3.2 Choice of agonist maintenance treatment	29
	6.3.3 Initial doses of opioid agonist maintenance treatment	32
	6.3.4 Fixed or flexible dosing in agonist maintenance treatment	32
	6.3.5 Maintenance doses of methadone	33
	6.3.6 Maintenance doses of buprenorphine	34
	6.3.7 Supervision of dosing in opioid agonist maintenance treatment	35
	6.3.8 Optimal duration of opioid agonist treatment	36
	6.3.9 Use of psychosocial interventions in maintenance treatment	37
6.4	Management of opioid withdrawal	38
	6.4.1 Signs, severity and treatment principles	38
	6.4.2 Assessment of opioid withdrawal	38
	6.4.3 Choice of treatments for assisting withdrawal from opioids	39
	6.4.4 Accelerated withdrawal management techniques	41
	6.4.5 Treatment setting for opioid withdrawal	43
	6.4.8 Psychosocial assistance in addition to pharmacological assistance for opioid withdrawal	44
6.5	Opioid antagonist (naltrexone) treatment	45
	6.5.1 Indications for opioid antagonist therapy	45
	6.5.2 Indications for naltrexone therapy	46
6.6	Psychosocial interventions	47
	6.6.1 Psychological interventions	47
	6.6.2 Social interventions	48
	6.6.3 Provision of psychosocial support	48
6.7	Treatment of overdose	48

6.8 Special considerations for specific groups and settings..49
   6.8.1 Patients with HIV/AIDS, hepatitis and TB..49
   6.8.2 Adolescents...49
   6.8.3 Women..51
   6.8.4 Pregnancy and breastfeeding...51
   6.8.5 Opium users..52
   6.8.6 Driving and operating machinery...52
   6.8.7 Psychiatric comorbidity with opioid dependence..52
   6.8.8 Polysubstance dependence..52
6.9 Management of pain in patients with opioid dependence..53
   6.9.1 Acute pain...53
   6.9.2 Chronic pain..54

Annex 1 Evidence profiles..55
Annex 2 Dispensing, dosing and prescriptions..70
Annex 3 ICD-10 codes for conditions covered in these guidelines...71
Annex 4 Pharmacology of medicines available for the treatment of opioid dependence................................72
Annex 5 Drug interactions involving methadone and buprenorphine..74
Annex 6 Alternatives for the treatment of opioid dependence not included in the current guidelines............77
Annex 7 Methadone and buprenorphine and international drug control conventions....................................78
Annex 8 Priorities for research...82
Annex 9 Background papers prepared for technical expert meetings to inform guideline development........84
Annex 10 Opioid withdrawal scales..85
Annex 11 Summary of characteristics of selected psychoactive substances..89
Annex 12 Prescribing guidelines..90
Annex 13 Glossary..93

References..96

Acknowledgements

These guidelines were produced by the World Health Organization (WHO), Department of Mental Health and Substance Abuse, in collaboration with the United Nations Office on Drugs and Crime (UNODC) a Guidelines Development Group of technical experts, and in consultation with the International Narcotics Control Board (INCB) secretariat and other WHO departments. WHO also wishes to acknowledge the financial contribution of UNODC and the Joint United Nations Programme on HIV/AIDS (UNAIDS) to this project.

GUIDELINES DEVELOPMENT GROUP

Marina Davoli
 Coordinating Editor
 Cochrane Review Group on Drugs and Alcohol
 Department of Epidemiology
 Osservatorio Epidemiologico Regione Lazio
 Roma
 Italy

Michael Farrell
 Reader/Consultant Psychiatrist
 National Addiction Centre
 Institute of Psychiatry and the Maudsley Hospital
 London
 United Kingdom

David Fiellin
 Associate Professor of Medicine
 Yale University School of Medicine
 United States of America

Li Jianhua
 Deputy Director
 Yunnan Institute for Drug Abuse
 China

Ratna Mardiati
 Psychiatrist
 Directorate General for Medical Care
 Jakarta
 Indonesia

Richard Mattick
 Director
 National Drug and Alcohol Research Centre
 University of New South Wales
 Sydney
 Australia

Elena Medina-Mora
 Director
 Epidemiology and Psychosocial Research
 National Institute of Psychiatry
 Mexico

Fred Owiti
 Consultant Psychiatrist
 Arrow Medical Centre
 Nairobi
 Kenya

Afarin Rahimi-Movaghar
 Iranian National Center for Addiction Studies
 Tehran University of Medical Sciences
 Tehran
 Iran

Rajat Ray
 Chief
 National Drug Dependence Treatment Centre
 All India Institute of Medical Sciences
 New Delhi
 India

Anthony J Smith
 Emeritus Professor
 Clinical Pharmacology
 Newcastle Mater Hospital
 Australia

Emilis Subata
 Director
 Vilnius Center for Addictive Disorders
 Lithuania

Ambros Uchtenhagen
 President
 Research Institute for Public Health and Addiction
 Zurich
 Switzerland

OBSERVERS

Council of Europe
Gabrielle Welle-Strand
Senior Adviser
Norwegian Directorate for Health and Social Affairs
Norway

International Narcotics Control Board Secretariat
Pavel Pachta
Chief, Narcotics Control and Estimates Section
Vienna
Austria

Carmen Selva-Bartolome
Chief, Psychotropics Control Section (until September 2007)
Vienna
Austria

Margarethe Ehrenfeldner
Chief, Psychotropics Control Section (as of 1 October 2007)
Vienna
Austria

UNITED NATIONS OFFICE ON DRUGS AND CRIME SECRETARIAT

Juana Tomas-Rossello
Drug Abuse Treatment Adviser, Global Challenges Section
Vienna
Austria

WORLD HEALTH ORGANIZATION SECRETARIAT

Department of Mental Health and Substance Abuse
Vladimir Poznyak
Co-ordinator

Nicolas Clark
Medical Officer

Hannu Alho
Temporary Advisor (seconded from the National Public Health Institute of Finland [KTL])

Department of HIV
Annette Verster
Technical Officer

Department of Health Systems Financing
Dan Chisholm
Economist

Department of Medicines Policy and Standards
Sue Hill
Medical Officer

Nicola Magrini
Medical Officer

Other contributors

WHO would also like to acknowledge the contribution made by the following individuals in the development of background materials and peer review:

Laura Amato, Department of Epidemiology, Azienda Sanitaria Locale "E", Rome, Italy

Mike Ashton, Drug and Alcohol Findings, United Kingdom

Anna Maria Bargagli, Department of Epidemiology, Azienda Sanitaria Locale "E", Rome, Italy

James Bell, National Addiction Centre, London, United Kingdom

Adrian Carter, Queensland Brain Institute, University of Queensland, Australia

Zhang Cunmin, Yunnan Institute for Drug Abuse, Kunming, Yunnan, China

Chris Doran, National Drug & Alcohol Research Centre, University of New South Wales, Australia

Colin Drummond, St George's, University of London, United Kingdom

Ralph Edwards, Director, Uppsala Monitoring Centre, Sweden

Gabriele Fischer, Medical University of Vienna, Austria

Andy Gray, University of KwaZulu-Natal, Durban, South Africa

Wayne Hall, School of Population Health, University of Queensland, Australia

S Kattimani, National Drug Dependence Treatment Centre, All India Institute of Medical Sciences, New Delhi, India

Nina Kopf, Department of Psychiatry, Medical University of Vienna, Austria

T Ladjevic, Research Institute for Public Health and Addiction, Zurich University, Switzerland

Lisa Marsch, Center for Drug Use and HIV Research, National Development and Research Institutes, New York, USA

Silvia Minozzi, Department of Epidemiology, Azienda Sanitaria Locale "E", Rome, Italy

Lubomir Okruhlica, Institute for Drug Dependencies, Centre for Treatment of Drug Dependencies, Bratislava, Slovak Republic

Katherine Perryman, St George's, University of London, United Kingdom

Carlo Perucci, Department of Epidemiology, Azienda Sanitaria Locale "E", Rome, Italy

Li Peikai, Yunnan Institute for Drug Abuse, Kunming, Yunnan, China

Jurgen Rehm, Research Institute for Public Health and Addiction, Zurich University, Centre for Addiction and Mental Health, Toronto, Canada

H K Sharma, National Drug Dependence Treatment Centre, All India Institute of Medical Sciences, New Delhi, India

Simona Vecchi, Department of Epidemiology, Azienda Sanitaria Locale "E", Rome, Italy

Declaration of interests of the guidelines development group

Michael Farrell reported being a member of the National Guidelines Group on Substance Dependence in the United Kingdom, receiving travel support and expenses for speaking at meetings from Reckitt Benckiser and Schering Plough (value <$1000 each occasion), and in collaboration with the University of Adelaide and the University of California, Los Angeles, receiving an unrestricted educational grant from Reckitt Benckiser (through the University of Adelaide) to organize a meeting on substance dependence in South East Asia, with no personal payments from the grant.

David Fiellin reported providing expert opinion at a congressional press conference related to treatment of substance dependence, and providing an expert review of methadone, buprenorphine and buprenorphine/naloxone for the United States Centre for Substance Abuse treatment, with no honorariums.

Richard Mattick reported providing advice and public statements on treatment of substance dependence in his role as Director of the National Drug and Alcohol Research Centre, receiving research support to his research unit as an untied educational grant from Reckitt Benckiser (value approximately $AU400 000 over 3 years), but without personal payment, and receiving research support to his research unit from the Australian National Health and Medical Research Council for research on substance dependence (value approximately $AU150 000).

Rajat Ray reported being a member of the Indian Expert Group for the Ministry of Health, India, on opioid substitution treatment and presenting a scientific paper on the topic in 2005, receiving funding for his research unit from Rusan Pharmaceuticals (value $US350 000) for research related to buprenorphine, with no personal payments.

Ambrose Uchtenhagen reported receiving funding for a literature review at least 3 years ago from Schering Plough.

Marina Davoli, Ratna Mardiati, Afarin Rahimi Movaghar, Fred Owiti, Emilis Subata, Anthony Smith, and Gabrielle Welle-Strand reported no conflict of interest.

Organizations providing feedback on the draft guidelines

- WHO Regional Offices
- WHO Collaborating Centres
  - Addiction Research Institute, Zurich, Switzerland
  - Centre for Addiction and Mental Health, Toronto, Canada
  - College on Problems of Drug Dependence, Vermont, Unites States
  - Drug and Alcohol Services Council, Adelaide, Australia
  - Institute of Health Science Research, Bangkok, Thailand
  - Mental Health Institute, Hunan, China
  - National Drug Research Institute, Perth, Australia
- Other organizations
  - American Association for the Treatment of Opioid Dependence
  - American College of Neuropsychopharmacology
  - American Society of Addiction Medicine
  - International Harm Reduction Association
  - International Center for Advancement of Addiction Treatment (ICAAT)
  - National Alliance of Methadone Advocates, New York, United States
  - National Institute on Drug Abuse, United States
  - National Institute for Health and Clinical Excellence (NICE), United Kingdom
  - Quest for Quality, the Netherlands
  - Service d'Abus de Substances, Département de Psychiatrie, Genève
  - South African National Council on Alcohol and Drug Dependence
  - Turning Point Alcohol & Drug Centre, Melbourne, Australia
  - World Psychiatric Association
  - South African National Council on Alcohol and Drug Dependence
  - Turning Point Alcohol & Drug Centre, Melbourne, Australia
  - World Psychiatric Association

Abbreviations and acronyms

6-MAM	6-monoacetylmorphine
AIDS	acquired immunodeficiency syndrome
ALT	alanine aminotransferase
AST	aspartate aminotransferase
ART	antiretroviral therapy
cAMP	cyclic adenosine monophosphate
CBT	cognitive behavioural therapy
CD4	cluster of differentiation 4 (T cell marker)
CI	confidence interval
CM	contingency management
CND	Commission on Narcotic Drugs
COWS	Clinical Opiate Withdrawal Scale
CPS	controlled prospective study
ECOSOC	United National Economic and Social Council
GABA	gamma-aminobutyric acid
GCMS	gas-chromatography and mass spectrometry
GDP	gross domestic product
HCV	hepatitis C virus
HIV	human immunodeficiency virus
ICD-10	International Classification of Diseases, 10th edition
INCB	International Narcotics Control Board
ITT	intention to treat
IV	intravenous
LAAM	levo-alpha-acetylmethadol
NAS	neonatal abstinence syndrome
NSAIDs	non-steriodal anti-inflammatory drugs
OOWS	Objective Opiate Withdrawal Scale
RCT	randomized controlled trial
RR	relative risk
SMD	standardized mean difference
SOWS	Subjective Opiate Withdrawal Scale
TB	Tuberculosis
UNAIDS	The Joint United Nations Programme on HIV/AIDS
UNODC	United Nations Office on Drugs and Crime
UROD	ultra-rapid opioid detoxification
WHO	World Health Organization
UN	United Nations

Executive summary

BACKGROUND TO THE DEVELOPMENT OF THESE GUIDELINES

These guidelines were developed in response to a resolution from the United Nations Economic and Social Council (ECOSOC), which invited the World Health Organization (WHO), in collaboration with the United Nations Office on Drugs and Crime (UNODC), "to develop and publish minimum requirements and international guidelines on psychosocially assisted pharmacological treatment of persons dependent on opioids"[1]. In accordance with WHO policy, the recommendations in these guidelines are based on systematic reviews of the available literature and consultation with a range of experts from different regions of the world. The GRADE evidence tables summarizing these reviews are contained in Annex 1 of this document.

INTENDED READERSHIP OF THESE GUIDELINES

These guidelines are intended to be read by those involved in providing psychosocially assisted pharmacological treatments at any level. The readership falls into three broad groups:
- policy makers and administrators who make decisions on the availability of medicines and the structure and funding of services in countries or in subnational health administrative regions
- managers and clinical leaders responsible for the organization of specific health-care services, and for the clinical care those services provide
- health-care workers treating patients within the health-care system.

EPIDEMIOLOGY OF OPIOID DEPENDENCE

UNODC estimates that there are 25 million problem drug users in world, of whom 15.6 are problem opioid users and 11.1 problem heroin users (approximately 0.3% of the global population)[2].[^1]

The global epidemic of HIV and acquired immune deficiency syndrome (AIDS) is often fuelled and maintained by unsafe injection practices, with an estimated 30% of new cases of HIV outside sub-Saharan Africa due to unsafe injecting,[5] particularly unsafe opioid injecting. The cost of this epidemic is counted in the millions of lives lost each year and the billions of dollars spent[6]. A comprehensive package of interventions to prevent the transmission of HIV must include measures to reduce unsafe injecting of opioids, including the treatment of opioid dependence[7,11].

As with other chronic conditions, opioid dependence tends mostly to follow a relapsing and remitting course.

PSYCHOSOCIALLY ASSISTED PHARMACOLOGICAL TREATMENTS

Psychosocially assisted pharmacological treatment refers to the combination of specific pharmacological and psychosocial measures used to reduce both illicit opioid use and harms related to opioid use and improve quality of life. While the psychosocial measures are varied, only a few specific medications are used for the treatment of opioid dependence.

Opioid agonist maintenance treatment is defined as the administration of thoroughly evaluated opioid agonists, by accredited professionals, in the framework of recognized medical practice, to people with opioid dependence, for achieving defined treatment aims[8,9,10]. Both methadone and buprenorphine are sufficiently long acting to be taken once daily under supervision, if necessary. When taken on a daily basis they do not produce the cycles of intoxication and withdrawal seen with shorter acting opioids, such as heroin. Both methadone and buprenorphine can also be used in reducing doses to assist in withdrawal from opioids, a process also referred to as opioid detoxification. Methadone and buprenorphine have a strong evidence base for their use, and have been placed on the WHO model list of essential medicines[8].

A different approach is that of assisting people dependent on opioids to withdraw from opioids completely, a process also referred to as opioid detoxification. Both methadone and buprenorphine can also be used in reducing doses to assist in withdrawal from opioids.

[^1]: The category of "problem drug user" is generally defined to include both dependent users and non dependent drug injectors.

Alpha-2 adrenergic agonists – such as clonidine – can also be used for opioid detoxification, to reduce the severity of opioid withdrawal symptoms.

Following detoxification, the long-acting opioid antagonist naltrexone can be used to prevent relapse to opioids. Naltrexone produces no opioid effects itself, and blocks the effects of opioids for 24–48 hours.

The short-acting opioid antagonist naloxone can be used to reverse the effects of opioid intoxication and overdose.

SUMMARY OF EVIDENCE AND RECOMMENDATIONS OF THESE GUIDELINES

Opioid agonist maintenance treatment

Of the treatment options examined, opioid agonist maintenance treatment, combined with psychosocial assistance, was found to be the most effective.

Oral methadone liquid and sublingual buprenorphine tablets are the medications most widely used for opioid agonist maintenance treatment. In the context of high-quality, supervised and well-organized treatment services, these medications interrupt the cycle of intoxication and withdrawal, greatly reducing heroin and other illicit opioid use, crime and the risk of death through overdose.

Compared to detoxification or no treatment, methadone maintenance treatment (using mostly supervised administration of the liquid methadone formulation) significantly reduces opioid and other drug use, criminal activity, HIV risk behaviours and transmission, opioid overdose and all-cause mortality; it also helps to retain people in treatment.

Compared to detoxification or no treatment, buprenorphine also significantly reduces drug use and improves treatment retention.

Methadone compared to buprenorphine for opioid agonist maintenance treatment

Comparing the evidence from clinical trials on the effectiveness of methadone and buprenorphine for opioid agonist maintenance treatment, both medications provide good outcomes in most cases. In general, methadone is recommended over buprenorphine, because it is more effective and costs less. However, buprenorphine has a slightly different pharmacological action; thus, making both medications available may attract greater numbers of people to treatment and may improve treatment matching.

Use of methadone in maintenance treatment

The initial methadone dose should be 20mg or less, depending on the level of opioid tolerance, allowing a high margin of safety to reduce inadvertent overdose. The dosage should be then quickly adjusted upwards if there are ongoing opioid withdrawal symptoms and downwards if there is any sedation. From there, the dose should be gradually increased to the point where illicit opioid use ceases; this is likely to be in the range of 60–120 mg methadone per day. Methadone use should be supervised initially. The degree of supervision should be individually tailored, and in accordance with local regulations; it should balance the benefits of reduced dosing frequency in stable patients with the risks of injection and diversion of methadone to the illicit drug market. Patients should be monitored with clinical assessment and drug testing. Psychosocial assistance should be offered to all patients.

Use of buprenorphine in maintenance treatment

Buprenorphine maintenance treatment should commence with a dose that is tailored to the pattern of opioid use, including the level of tolerance, the duration of action of opioids used and the timing of most recent opioid use (usually 4mg). From there, the dose should be rapidly increased (i.e. over days) to one that produces stable effects for 24 hours; this is generally in the range of 8–24 mg buprenorphine per day. Generally, if there is continuing opioid use, the dose should be increased. Dosing supervision and other aspects of treatment should be determined on an individual basis, using the same criteria as for methadone maintenance treatment.

Treatment for withdrawal and prevention of relapse

Opioid withdrawal (rather than maintenance treatment) results in poor outcomes in the long term; however, patients should be helped to withdraw from opioids if it is their informed choice to do so. Withdrawal from opioids can be conducted either on an outpatient or an inpatient basis, using reducing doses of methadone or buprenorphine, or alpha-2 agonists. Methadone and buprenorphine are the preferred treatments for opioid withdrawal, because they are effective and can be used in a supervised fashion in both inpatient and outpatient settings. Inpatient treatment is more effective, but it is also more expensive and is recommended only for a minority of patients (e.g. those with polysubstance dependence, or medical or psychiatric comorbidity). Accelerated withdrawal techniques using opioid antagonists in combination with heavy sedation are not recommended because of safety concerns.

Use of naltrexone to prevent relapse

Naltrexone can be useful in preventing relapse in those who have withdrawn from opioids, particularly in those who are already motivated to abstain from opioid use. Following opioid withdrawal, patients who are motivated to abstain from opioid use should be advised to consider naltrexone to prevent relapse.

PSYCHOSOCIAL TREATMENT

Psychosocial interventions – including cognitive and behavioural approaches and contingency management techniques – can add to the effectiveness of treatment, if combined with agonist maintenance treatment and medications for assisting opioid withdrawal. Psychosocial services should be made available to all patients, although those who do not take up the offer should not be denied effective pharmacological treatment.

TREATMENT SYSTEMS

In planning treatment systems, resources should be distributed in a way that delivers effective treatment to as many people as possible. Opioid agonist maintenance treatment appears to be the most cost-effective treatment, and should therefore form the backbone of the treatment system for opioid dependence. Countries with established opioid agonist maintenance programmes usually attract 40–50% of dependent opioid users into such programmes, with higher rates in some urban environments. Because of their cost, inpatient facilities should be reserved for those with specific needs, and most patients wanting to withdraw from opioids should be encouraged to attempt opioid withdrawal as outpatients.

ETHICAL PRINCIPLES OF CARE

When treating people with opioid dependence, ethical principles should be considered, together with evidence from clinical trials; the human rights of opioid-dependent individuals should always be respected. Treatment decisions should be based on standard principles of medical-care ethics – providing equitable access to treatment and psychosocial support that best meets the needs of the individual patient. Treatment should respect and validate the autonomy of the individual, with patients being fully informed about the risks and benefits of treatment choices. Furthermore, programmes should create supportive environments and relationships to facilitate treatment, provide coordinated treatment of comorbid mental and physical disorders, and address relevant psychosocial factors.

RECOMMENDATIONS

This section lists all the recommendations contained in these guidelines.

Recommendations for action at policy or health-system levels are marked as either marked "minimal" or "best practice":
- *minimal* recommendations are suggested for adoption in all settings as a minimum standard; these should be considered the minimal requirements for the provision of treatment of opioid dependence
- *best practice* recommendations represent preferred strategies for achieving the optimal public health benefit in the provision of treatment for opioid dependence.

The document contains recommendations based on evidence from systematic reviews and meta-analyses, taking into consideration evidence from other sources, technical considerations, resource implications and the risks and benefits of different alternatives. As recommended in the GRADE system, recommendations were divided into two strengths, here termed as "strong" or "standard" recommendations.

- *strong* recommendations are those for which:
  - most individuals should receive the intervention, assuming that they have been informed about and understand its benefits, harms and burdens
  - most individuals would want the recommended course of action and only a small proportion would not
  - the recommendation could unequivocally be used for policy making
- *standard* recommendations are those for which:
  - most individuals would want the suggested course of action, but an appreciable proportion would not
  - values and preferences vary widely
- policy making will require extensive debates and involvement of many stakeholders.

Some recommendations do not include an indication of strength – this means that the recommendation was ungraded.

Summary of recommendations

Recommendations for health systems at national and subnational levels		
	Minimal requirements	**Best practice**
Treatment strategy		A strategy document should be produced outlining the government policy on the treatment of opioid dependence. The strategy should aim for adequate coverage, quality and safety of treatment.
Legal framework	Psychosocially assisted pharmacological treatment should not be compulsory.	
Treatment funding and availability	Treatment should be accessible to disadvantaged populations. Pharmacological treatment of opioid dependence should be widely accessible; this might include treatment delivery in primary care settings. Patients with comorbidities can be treated in primary health-care settings if there is access to specialist consultation when necessary. At the time of commencement of a treatment service, there should be a realistic prospect of that service being financially viable. Essential pharmacological treatment options should consist of opioid agonist maintenance treatment and services for the management of opioid withdrawal. At a minimum, this would include either methadone or buprenorphine for opioid agonist maintenance and outpatient withdrawal management.	To achieve optimal coverage and treatment outcomes, treatment of opioid dependence should be provided free of charge, or covered by public health-care insurance. Pharmacological treatment of opioid dependence should be accessible to all those in need, including those in prison and other closed settings. Pharmacological treatment options should consist of both methadone and buprenorphine for opioid agonist maintenance and opioid withdrawal, alpha-2 adrenergic agonists for opioid withdrawal, naltrexone for relapse prevention, and naloxone for the treatment of overdose.

Recommendations for treatment programmes		
	Minimal requirements	**Best practice**
Clinical governance	Treatment services should have a system of clinical governance, with a chain of clinical accountability within the health-care system, to ensure that the minimal standards for provision of opioid dependence treatment are being met.	A process of clinical governance should be established to ensure that treatments for opioid dependence are both safe and effective. The process should be transparent and outlined in a clinical governance document. Treatment of opioid dependence should be provided within the health-care system.
Consent to treatment	Patients must give informed consent for treatment.	
Training of staff	Treatment of opioid dependence should be carried out by trained health-care personnel. The level of training for specific tasks should be determined by the level of responsibility and national regulations.	Health authorities should ensure that treatment providers have sufficient skills and qualifications to use controlled substances appropriately. These requirements may include postgraduate training and certification, continuing education and licensing, and the setting aside of funding for monitoring and evaluation.
Medical records	Up-to-date medical records should be kept for all patients. These should include, as a minimum, the history, clinical examination, investigations, diagnosis, health and social status, treatment plans and their revisions, referrals, evidence of consent, prescribed drugs and other interventions received. Confidentiality of patient records should be ensured. Health-care providers involved in the treatment of an individual should have access to patient data in accordance with national regulations, as should patients themselves. Health-care providers or other personnel involved in patient treatment should not share information about patients with police and other law enforcement authorities unless a patient approves, or unless required by law. Patients treated with opioid agonists should be identifiable to treating staff.	
Pharmacy records	Documented processes should be established to ensure the safe and legal procurement, storage, dispensing and dosing of medicines, particularly of methadone and buprenorphine.	
Clinical guidelines	Clinical guidelines for the treatment of opioid dependence should be available to clinical staff.	Clinical guidelines should be detailed, comprehensive, evidence based and developed at a country level or lower, to reflect local laws, policies and conditions.
Opioid agonist maintenance dosing policies	To maximize the safety and effectiveness of agonist maintenance treatment programmes, policies and regulations should encourage flexible dosing structures, with low starting doses and high maintenance doses, and without placing restrictions on dose levels and the duration of treatment.	

Recommendations for treatment programmes		
	Minimal requirements	**Best practice**
Detoxification services		Opioid withdrawal services should be structured such that withdrawal is not a stand-alone service but is integrated with ongoing treatment options.
Take home doses		Take-home doses can be recommended when the dose and social situation are stable, and when there is a low risk of diversion for illegitimate purposes.
Involuntary discharge		Involuntary discharge from treatment is justified to ensure the safety of staff and other patients, but noncompliance with programme rules alone should not generally be a reason for involuntary discharge. Before involuntary discharge, reasonable measures to improve the situation should be taken, including re-evaluation of the treatment approach used.
Assessment and choice of treatment	A detailed individual assessment should be conducted which includes: history (past treatment experiences; medical and psychiatric history; living conditions; legal issues; occupational situation; and social and cultural factors, that may influence substance use); clinical examination (assessment of intoxication / withdrawal, injection marks); and, if necessary, investigations (such as urine drug screen, HIV, Hep C, Hep B, TB, liver function). Urine drug testing should be available for use at initial assessment when a recent history of opioid use cannot be verified by other means (e.g. evidence of opioid withdrawal or intoxication).	The choice of treatment for an individual should be based on a detailed assessment of the treatment needs, appropriateness of treatment to meet those needs (assessment of appropriateness should be evidence based), patient acceptance and treatment availability. Screening for psychiatric and somatic comorbidity should form part of the initial assessment. Voluntary testing for HIV and common infectious diseases should be available as part of an individual assessment, accompanied by counselling before and after testing. Ideally, all patients should be tested at initial assessment for recent drug use. Treatment plans should take a long-term perspective. Opioid withdrawal should be planned in conjunction with ongoing treatment.
Range of services to be offered	Essential pharmacological treatment options should consist of opioid agonist maintenance treatment and services for the management of opioid withdrawal. Naloxone should be available for treating opioid overdose.	Pharmacological treatment options should consist of both methadone and buprenorphine for opioid agonist maintenance and opioid withdrawal, alpha-2 adrenergic agonists for opioid withdrawal, naltrexone for relapse prevention, and naloxone for the treatment of overdose.
Psychosocial support availability	Psychosocial support should be available to all opioid-dependent patients, in association with pharmacological treatments of opioid dependence. At a minimum, this should include assessment of psychosocial needs, supportive counselling and links to existing family and community services.	A variety of structured psychosocial interventions should be available, according to the needs of the patients. Such interventions may include - but are not limited to - different forms of counselling and psychotherapy, and assistance with social needs such as housing, employment, education, welfare and legal problems.

Recommendations for treatment programmes		
	Minimal requirements	**Best practice**
Availability of treatment for comorbid medical conditions	Links to HIV, hepatitis and TB treatment services (where they exist) should be provided.	Onsite psychosocial and psychiatric treatment should be provided for patients with psychiatric comorbidity.
		Where there are significant numbers of opioid-dependent patients with either HIV, hepatitis or TB, treatment of opioid dependence should be integrated with medical services for these conditions.
		For patients with TB, hepatitis or HIV and opioid dependence, opioid agonists should be administered in conjunction with medical treatment; there is no need to wait for abstinence from opioids to commence either anti-TB medication, treatment for hepatitis or antiretroviral medication.
		Opioid-dependent patients with TB, hepatitis or HIV should have equitable access to treatment for TB, hepatitis, HIV and opioid dependence.
Availability of hepatitis B vaccine		Treatment services should offer hepatitis B vaccination to all opioid-dependent patients.
Treatment evaluation	There should be a system for monitoring the safety of the treatment service, including the extent of medication diversion.	There should be intermittent or ongoing evaluation of both the process and outcomes of the treatment provided.

Recommendations for treatment of the individual patient		Strength of recommendation	Quality of evidence
Choice of treatment	For the pharmacological treatment of opioid dependence, clinicians should offer opioid withdrawal, opioid agonist maintenance and opioid antagonist (naltrexone) treatment, but most patients should be advised to use opioid agonist maintenance treatment.	Strong	Low to moderate
	For opioid-dependent patients not commencing opioid agonist maintenance treatment, consider antagonist pharmacotherapy using naltrexone following the completion of opioid withdrawal.	Standard	Low
Opioid agonist maintenance treatment	For opioid agonist maintenance treatment, most patients should be advised to use methadone in adequate doses in preference to buprenorphine.	Strong	High
	During methadone induction, the initial daily dose should depend on the level of neuroadaptation; it should generally not be more than 20 mg, and certainly not more than 30mg.	Strong	Very low
	On average, methadone maintenance doses should be in the range of 60–120 mg per day.	Strong	Low
	Average buprenorphine maintenance doses should be at least 8 mg per day.	Standard	Very low
	Methadone and buprenorphine doses should be directly supervised in the early phase of treatment.	Strong	Very low
	Take-away doses may be provided for patients when the benefits of reduced frequency of attendance are considered to outweigh the risk of diversion, subject to regular review.	Standard	Very low
	Psychosocial support should be offered routinely in association with pharmacological treatment for opioid dependence.	Strong	High
Management of opioid withdrawal	For the management of opioid withdrawal, tapered doses of opioid agonists should generally be used, although alpha-2 adrenergic agonists may also be used.	Standard	Moderate
	Clinicians should not routinely use the combination of opioid antagonists and minimal sedation in the management of opioid withdrawal.	Standard	Very low
	Clinicians should not use the combination of opioid antagonists with heavy sedation in the management of opioid withdrawal.	Strong	Low
	Psychosocial services should be routinely offered in combination with pharmacological treatment of opioid withdrawal.	Standard	Moderate
Pregnancy	Opioid agonist maintenance treatment should be used for the treatment of opioid dependence in pregnancy.	Strong	Very low
	Methadone maintenance should be used in pregnancy in preference to buprenorphine maintenance for the treatment of opioid dependence; although there is less evidence about the safety of buprenorphine, it might also be offered.	Standard	Very low

1 Scope and purpose

These guidelines have been developed in response to the resolution *Guidelines for psychosocially assisted pharmacological treatment of persons dependent on opioids* of the United Nations Economic and Social Council (ECOSOC). The resolution invited the World Health Organization (WHO), in collaboration with United Nations Office on Drugs and Crime (UNODC), "to develop and publish minimum requirements and international guidelines on psychosocially assisted pharmacological treatment of persons dependent on opioids, taking into account regional developments in the field, in order to assist the member states concerned"[1].

These guidelines are intended to be read by those involved in providing psychosocially assisted pharmacological treatment of opioid dependence at any level. Chapter 2 explains how the guidelines were formulated, and Chapter 3 provides background information on opioid dependence. Chapters 4–6 are directed, respectively, at the three broad groups for whom this document is intended:
- policy makers and administrators who make decisions on the availability of medicines, and on the structure and funding of services in countries or in subnational health administrative regions
- managers and clinical leaders responsible for the organization of specific health-care services, and for the clinical care those services provide
- health-care workers treating patients within the health-care system.

National and regional programmes, and treatment guideline groups may wish to use this document to assist in the development of locally adapted guidelines.

The clinical questions addressed by these guidelines were developed in consultation with clinicians and academics from various countries involved in the management of opioid dependence. The questions addressed by these guidelines can be summarized briefly as:
- What medications should be used for the management of opioid dependence and withdrawal? Further questions related to this issue are:
  - Should preference be given to opioid agonist maintenance treatment, detoxification or antagonist treatment?
  - Which medications should be used for each approach?
  - How should medications be administered (optimal dose, level of dosing supervision, etc.)?
- What level and type of psychosocial support should be provided to opioid-dependent patients?
- What specific treatment should be offered to specific groups (e.g. people with human immunodeficiency virus (HIV) and pregnant women)?
- What are the minimal standards for provision of treatment for opioid dependence?

The recommendations in the guidelines operate at three levels:
- treatment systems at national and subnational levels (policy, legislation, funding, regional and country planning) (see Chapter 4)
- treatment programmes (methods of organization and provision of care) (see Chapter 5)
- treatment of the individual patient (see Chapter 6).

Recommendations made at the level of the individual patient are based on systematic reviews of clinical trials, summarized in Annex 1. Recommendations at the other two levels are based on a range of evidence, including extrapolation of clinical trial data by experts in the guidelines development group, epidemiological studies and the principles of medical ethics.

The medications considered in these guidelines are methadone, buprenorphine, naltrexone and adrenergic alpha-2 agonists (clonidine, lofexidine and guanfacine). Although other medications show promise in the treatment of opioid dependence, they have not been included in these guidelines because there is insufficient evidence to make a full analysis of their effectiveness; thus, including them would significantly increase the complexity of the guidelines. A brief description of the pharmacology of these medications is included in Annex 4.

The aims of these guidelines are to:
- reduce global barriers to the effective treatment of opioid dependence
- contribute to the development of evidence-based and ethical treatment policies for opioid

dependence
- contribute to improvement of the quality of pharmacological treatment of opioid dependence
- facilitate implementation of effective treatment policies and programmes for opioid dependence.

The guidelines are not:
- a comprehensive guide to opioid dependence or its treatment
- a replacement for clinical judgement
- a description of local regulations for the provision of opioid dependence treatment.

The guidelines cover not only opioid dependence, but also treatment of opioid overdose and opioid withdrawal.

2   Method of formulating recommendations

The *WHO Guidelines for the Psychosocially Assisted Pharmacological Treatment of Opioid Dependence* were prepared according to the WHO *Guidelines for WHO Guidelines* (2003)[12], modified as necessary to provide advice:
- on many complex clinical questions for which evidence is lacking
- even in the absence of high-quality evidence.

A group of technical experts – international scientists with expertise in opioid dependence and clinical guidelines development – was convened in 2005, and again in 2006 and 2007. The membership of this group is detailed in the acknowledgements section. In their first meeting, the group defined the key questions to be addressed by the guidelines. For each key clinical question, the literature was searched for recent systematic reviews on the topic. Where a Cochrane review[2] existed, that review was used in preference to other reviews. Where no suitable systematic review existed, a review was conducted.

At its meeting in 2006, the group assessed the evidence and formulated recommendations. The quality of the evidence was assessed according to the methodology described by the GRADE working group[13]. This approach involves assessing the quality of evidence on a particular question, taking into consideration the magnitude of the effect, the relevance of the data to the clinical question being asked, the sample size in the relevant trials, the methodology of the trials and the consistency of the findings. At the start of this process, each health outcome was rated from 1 to 9, according to its importance. The GRADE convention on the rating of outcomes is as follows:
- ratings of 7–9 are for critical health outcomes
- ratings of 4–6 are for outcomes that are considered important but not critical to the decision; they should be used in judgements about tradeoffs and recommendations, but not in judgements about the overall quality of evidence across critical outcomes
- ratings of 1–3 are generally removed from the evidence profile and are not considered in judgements about the overall quality of evidence, tradeoffs or recommendations.

In some instances, additional meta-analyses were conducted from the systematic review data:
- to exclude non-randomized controlled trials (non-RCTs) (where Cochrane reviews had included non-randomized trials)
- to reverse some outcomes and thus maintain outcome consistency (e.g. using "drop out" as the primary outcome measure of retention rather than "still in treatment")
- to reverse the order of the comparisons, where necessary (e.g. methadone versus buprenorphine instead of buprenorphine versus methadone).
- to examine an additional outcome of interest (e.g. the addition of seroconversion as an outcome measure in the review of opioid agonist treatment and HIV).

In the GRADE system, evidence is classified as "high", "moderate", "low" or "very low". Definitions are as follows:
- *High* – Further research is very unlikely to change confidence in the estimate of effect.
- *Moderate* – Further research is likely to have an important impact on confidence in the estimate of effect and may change the estimate.
- *Low* – Further research is very likely to have an important impact on confidence in the estimate of effect and is likely to change the estimate.
- *Very low* – Any estimate of effect is very uncertain.

The resulting evidence profiles are listed in Annex 1.

To produce a series of recommendations, the technical experts considered the evidence from these reviews and meta-analyses, taking into consideration evidence from other sources, technical considerations, resource implications and the risks and benefits of different alternatives.

The strength of each recommendation is based on considerations of the effectiveness of the intervention, the strength of the evidence, the resource implications,

---
2   http://www.cochrane.org/

the balance between benefits and harms, and a consideration of ethical implications. As recommended in the GRADE system, recommendations are divided into two strengths, here termed as "strong" or "standard" recommendations.

"Strong" recommendations can be interpreted as follows:
- Most individuals should receive the intervention, assuming that they have been informed about and understand its benefits, harms and burdens.
- Most individuals would want the recommended course of action and only a small proportion would not.
- The recommendation could unequivocally be used for policy making.

"Standard" recommendations can be interpreted as follows:
- Most individuals would want the suggested course of action, but an appreciable proportion would not.
- Values and preferences vary widely.
- Policy making will require extensive debates and involvement of many stakeholders.

Some recommendations do not include an indication of strength – this means that the recommendation is ungraded.

A draft of the guidelines was circulated for feedback in July 2007 to selected organizations, WHO departments and regional offices, and WHO collaborating centres; it was also provided to individuals on request. This draft, along with received submissions, was considered at the third meeting in September 2007.

These guidelines are likely to require updating in the near future, given the pace of research in this field, the multitude of alternative treatments not considered here and the relatively scant published experience to date in less resourced countries. The recommendations are therefore expected to remain valid for the next three years only.

The WHO Department of Mental Health and Substance Abuse will take responsibility for updating these guidelines.

Policy and programme-level recommendations are based on the evidence from the GRADE process, combined with other evidence not reviewed systematically, including the opinion of the members of the technical expert group. Consequently, there are no GRADE tables corresponding to the recommendations in these sections.

2.1 Conventions for reporting clinical trial data

Clinical trial data are summarized in these guidelines. When comparing outcomes classed as categorical variables (e.g. mortality, retention in treatment or abstinence from opioids), the relative risk is used (RR). The relative risk is the ratio of the probability of a particular outcome in the population exposed to a particular intervention or risk factor, compared to the probability of that outcome occurring without exposure to the risk factor or intervention. For example, if an RCT compared a group of heroin users on methadone with a group assigned to detoxification, and found that those in the methadone group had a relative risk of heroin use of 0.32, this would mean that, on average, people with opioid dependence are approximately one third as likely to be using heroin if they are treated with methadone than if they undergo opioid detoxification.

For continuous variables (e.g. the severity of opioid withdrawal, or the number of opioid-positive urine tests for each study participant), the standardized mean difference (SMD) or weighted mean difference is used with a meta-analysis. The standardised mean difference, used for non-comparable scales, is the difference between two means, divided by an estimate of the within-group standard deviation. The weighted mean difference is used for comparable scales.

The 95% confidence interval (CI) for a relative risk or mean difference expresses the range that is highly likely (i.e. 19 times out of 20) to contain the true relative risk or mean difference, based on the data available. For example, the 95% confidence interval for the relative risk of dying in the follow-up period if randomly allocated to methadone compared to detoxification is 0.29 to 0.48; this implies that there is a 95% chance that the true relative risk lies in this range.

3 Background

3.1 Opioid dependence

Opioid dependence is characterized by a cluster of cognitive, behavioural and physiological features. The *International Classification of Diseases, 10th edition* (ICD-10)[14] identifies six such features:
- a strong desire or sense of compulsion to take opioids
- difficulties in controlling opioid use
- a physiological withdrawal state
- tolerance
- progressive neglect of alternative pleasures or interests because of opioid use
- persisting with opioid use despite clear evidence of overtly harmful consequences.

ICD-10 defines opioid dependence as the "presence of three of more [of these features] present simultaneously at any one time in the preceding year" (see Annex 3 for more details).

Opioid dependence does not develop without a period of regular use, although regular use alone is not sufficient to induce dependence.

3.2 Neurobiological aspects of opioid dependence

Repeated opioid use induces a series of neuroadaptations in various neuronal circuits in the brain that are involved in motivation, memory, behaviour control and disinhibition. The result is an increased and long-lasting reward value associated with the use of opioids and the environmental cues associated with such use, and a decreased reward value associated with natural reinforcers encountered in everyday life events[15].

Recent decades have seen a substantial increase in our understanding of the neurobiological aspects of substance dependence[9]. We now know that certain parts of the brain have an important role in regulating pleasurable behaviours, and that neuronal pathways to and from these areas form so-called "reward circuits". They are located within the mesocorticolimbic dopamine systems originating in the ventral tegmental area, projecting to the nucleus accumbens, amygdala, and prefrontal cortex area[16].

In the 1970s and 1980s, the existence of multiple opioid receptors was reported, and further pharmacological research suggested the classification of opioid binding sites into three receptor classes, referred to as mu, delta and kappa receptors[17, 18]. Since then, our understanding has further developed and we now know that opioid receptors belong to the family of G-protein coupled receptors, and that each receptor class has several subtypes[19].

The opioid effects of analgesia, euphoria and sedation are mediated primarily by the mu receptor. Opioids induce dopamine release indirectly by decreasing gamma-aminobutyric acid (GABA) inhibition via mu receptors in the ventral tegmental area[20, 21, 22]. They also induce dopamine release directly, by interacting with opioid receptors in the nucleus accumbens[23, 24].

The effect of chronic opioid exposure on opioid receptor levels has not been well defined in humans. Tolerance develops through multiple mechanisms, including an acute desensitization of the opioid receptor (which develops within minutes of opioid use and resolves within hours after use), and a long-term desensitization of the opioid receptor (which persists for several days after removal of opioid agonists). Changes also occur in the number of opioid receptors[25], and there is compensatory up-regulation of the cyclic adenosine monophosphate (cAMP) producing enzymes. When the opioid is withdrawn, the cAMP cascade becomes overactive, leading to the "noradrenergic storm" seen clinically as opioid withdrawal, which may create a drive to reinstate substance use. The intensely dysphoric withdrawal syndrome is characterized by watery eyes, runny nose, yawning, sweating, restlessness, irritability, tremor, nausea, vomiting, diarrhoea, increased blood pressure, chills, cramps and muscles aches; it can last seven days or even longer.

Long-term changes in neuronal circuitry, similar to those seen in learning and memory, can occur as a result of repeated opioid use. This effect creates a high risk of relapse to opioid use even after long periods of abstinence[26].

3.3 Epidemiology of illicit opioid use and dependence

Opioid dependence is a worldwide health problem that has enormous economic, personal and public health consequences. There are an estimated 15.6 million illicit opioid users in the world, of whom 11 million use heroin[2]. Opioids are the main drugs of abuse in Asia, Europe and much of Oceania, and it is estimated that globally the consumption of the opioid class of drugs is increasing[2].

3.4 Harms associated with opioid use

Injecting drug use has been strongly associated with HIV, accounting for 30% of HIV infections outside sub-Saharan Africa, and up to 80% of cases in some countries in eastern Europe and central Asia[5]. Once it enters a drug-using population, HIV can spread rapidly, and new epidemics of HIV infection mediated by intravenous drug use are occurring in sub-Saharan Africa[2]. Despite this situation, measures that prevent the spread of HIV in IDU, including opioid agonist maintenance treatment, have less than 5% coverage worldwide[27].

Unsafe injecting practices associated with injecting drug use have also led to a global epidemic of hepatitis C. An estimated 130 million people are infected with hepatitis C, with 3–4 million people newly infected each year[28]. Unsafe injection practices are the main route of transmission, accounting for an estimated 90% of new hepatitis C infections.

In countries with a low prevalence of HIV, opioid-dependent individuals have been found to have an annual mortality of 2–4% per annum, or 13 times that of their peers[29]. This increased mortality is primarily due to overdoses, violence, suicide, and smoking and alcohol-related causes[30, 31, 32]. In countries with high HIV prevalence, acquired immunodeficiency syndrome (AIDS) also makes a significant contribution to mortality[33].

Opioid dependence per se is associated with a significant reduction in quality of life as meaningful activities become replaced by time spent intoxicated or seeking opioids[34]. In addition to medical comorbidity associated with injecting drug use and violence, illicit opioid users have high rates of psychiatric comorbidity – in particular, depression and post-traumatic stress disorder[35].

3.5 Economic consequences of opioid use

Opioid dependence imposes a significant economic burden on society, not only in terms of directly attributable health-care costs (e.g. treatment and prevention services, and other health-care use), but also in terms of its impact on other budgets (notably social welfare and criminal justice services). Opioid dependence also has an effect on productivity, due to unemployment, absenteeism, and premature mortality.

Studies in industrialized countries have attempted to place an economic value on the aggregate impact of these consequences, with findings of from 0.2 to 2% of a country's gross domestic product (GDP)[36, 37, 38].

3.6 Natural history of opioid dependence

Cohort studies of dependent illicit opioid users show that although a significant proportion (10–40%) are abstinent at follow-up, most continue to use illicit opioids[39, 40, 41, 42]. Contact with treatment is one factor associated with recovery from opioid dependence; other factors include personal motivation, religion, spirituality, family and employment[41].

3.7 Opioid dependence as a medical condition

Historically, opioid dependence was often seen as a disorder of willpower, reflecting poorly on the character of an individual. However, with recent advances in the understanding of the biological mechanism behind dependence and its implications, it has now been widely accepted that, regardless of the reasons for opioid use, the neurological changes that occur with opioid dependence constitute a brain disorder. Therefore, opioid dependence can be considered as a medical condition, with complex sociological and individual determinants. Opioid dependence is characterized by a series of symptoms that have long-term prognostic implications, and for which treatment options now exist[9].

3.8 Treatment of opioid dependence

Treatment of opioid dependence is a set of pharmacological and psychosocial interventions aimed at:
- reducing or ceasing opioid use
- preventing future harms associated with opioid use
- improving quality of life and well-being of the opioid-dependent patient.

Treatment of drug dependence can serve a multitude of purposes. Beyond reductions in drug usage, it can help the drug user to see his or her problems from a different perspective, improve self-reliance, and empower the individual to seek and effect changes in their life; it can even confer self-esteem and give hope. At the same time, it can provide access to physical and psychiatric care and social assistance, and provide for the needs of the patient's family as well as those of the patient.

In most cases, treatment will be required in the long term or even throughout life. The aim of treatment services in such instances is not only to reduce or stop opioid use, but also to improve health and social functioning, and to help patients avoid some of the more serious consequences of drug use. Such long-term treatment, common for many medical conditions, should not be seen as treatment failure, but rather as a cost-effective way of prolonging life and improving quality of life, supporting the natural and long-term process of change and recovery.

Broadly speaking, there are two pharmacological approaches to opioid dependence treatment – those based on opioid withdrawal and those based on agonist maintenance.

3.8.1 MANAGEMENT OF OPIOID WITHDRAWAL

Pharmacological management of opioid withdrawal is usually by one of the following:
- gradual cessation of an opioid agonist (i.e. methadone)
- short-term use of a partial agonist (i.e. buprenorphine)
- sudden opioid cessation and use of alpha-2 adrenergic agonists to relieve withdrawal symptoms.

In practice, most patients resume opioid use within six months of commencing opioid withdrawal[43, 44]; the implication being that a single detoxification episode should not be promoted as effective treatment.

3.8.2 AGONIST MAINTENANCE TREATMENT

Agonist maintenance treatment usually consists of daily administration of an opioid agonist (e.g. methadone) or a partial agonist (e.g. buprenorphine). The resulting stable level of opioid effect is experienced by the dependent user as neither intoxication nor withdrawal, but more as "normal". The aims of agonist maintenance treatment include:
- reduction or cessation of illicit opioids
- reduction or cessation of injecting and associated risk of bloodborne virus transmission
- reduction of overdose risk
- reduction of criminal activity
- improvement in psychological and physical health.

In practice, most patients commencing opioid agonist treatment will cease heroin or use it infrequently, with only 20–30% reporting ongoing regular heroin use[43, 45]. However, relapse to heroin use following the cessation of agonist maintenance treatment is common[46, 47, 48] and research is lacking on when, who and how to withdraw from opioid agonist maintenance treatment.

3.8.4 PSYCHOSOCIAL ASSISTANCE

Psychosocial assistance in the treatment of opioid dependence refers to the many ways in which professional and non-professional members of society can support the psychological health and the social environment of the opioid user, to help improve both the quality and duration of life. Assistance can range from the simple (e.g. provision of food and shelter) to the complex (e.g. structured psychotherapy); this topic is discussed in Chapter 6.

4 Guidelines for health systems at national and subnational levels

The WHO constitution[49] defines health as "a state of complete physical, mental and social well-being and not merely the absence of disease or infirmity". It goes on to state that the enjoyment of the highest attainable standard of health is one of the fundamental rights of every human being, without distinction of race, religion, political belief, economic or social condition. The constitution also states that the health of all peoples is fundamental to the attainment of peace and security, and is dependent upon the fullest cooperation of individuals and states. Similarly, the Ottawa charter[50] outlines the link between health and broader social policy and health systems, highlighting the importance of actions at the health-system level.

These guidelines contain two levels of recommendations for action at the health-system level – "minimal" and "optimal". Recommendations marked "minimal" are suggested for adoption in all settings as a minimum standard; they should be considered the minimal requirements for the provision of treatment of opioid dependence. Recommendations marked "optimal" represent best practice strategies for achieving the maximal public health benefit in the provision of treatment for opioid dependence.

4.1 International regulations

Nations operate within an international regulatory framework; and methadone and buprenorphine are medicines under international control. The Single Convention on Narcotic Drugs, 1961 (as revised by the 1972 protocol) and the Convention on Psychotropic Substances, 1971, outline specific control requirements for those substances (details of requirements of these conventions are given in Annex 7). The conventions also include the requirement to make treatment available for people who are dependent upon narcotic drugs or psychotropic substances. The two main objectives of these conventions are to make narcotic drugs and psychotropic substances (including opioids) available for medical and scientific purposes, and to prevent their diversion for other purposes.

Responsible authorities should familiarise themselves with the international and legal regulations for the procurement, distribution, storage and prescription of opioids. If a country does not have regulations concerning the dispensing of agonist maintenance medications and provision of interventions, then these should be developed in accordance with the relevant conventions. The laws and regulations should enable prescribed methadone and buprenorphine to be dispensed – either under supervision or as take-home doses – from accessible dispensing points, while preventing diversion for non-medical use.

Treatment providers should familiarize themselves with the national and subnational requirements, and ensure that the treatment provided is consistent with relevant laws and regulations.

International agreements that outline responsibilities for the protection of human rights are also relevant to opioid treatment (see ethical issues, below).

4.2 Opioid dependence as a health-care issue

Substance dependence per se should be regarded as a health problem and not a legal one. Given the multiple medical problems associated with opioid dependence and the nature of pharmacological treatment, provision of pharmacological treatment for opioid dependence should be a health-care priority. This is encouraged in the Single Convention on Narcotic Drugs, 1961, which encourages parties to give special attention to, and take all practicable measures for, the prevention and treatment of the abuse of narcotic drugs. The convention also stipulates that treatment may be made available as an alternative to conviction or punishment (or in addition to them) to those people with substance-use disorders who have committed punishable offences.

4.3 National treatment policy

When a treatment system is developed in any country, it should be planned as part of the community's overall resources for dealing with health and social problems (WHO Expert Committee 30th Report).[10, 50]

The policy should outline the approach to preventing and treating the problems of opioid dependence. It should be based on epidemiological data, the evidence for effectiveness of interventions, the resources of the country and the values of the society.

Estimating treatment need is important for planning treatment services, and for reviewing the accessibility of services to different population groups. Estimating the number of opioid-dependent people in a population from household surveys is difficult due to their under representation in large-scale epidemiological surveys. Alternative techniques that can be more effective are capture–recapture, back projection and multiplier methods[51]. WHO has produced guidance on how to estimate the number of opioid-dependent people[52].

Treatment need can also be estimated using systems that monitor treatment, including the demand for first-time treatment. However, some populations may be underrepresented in estimates of those seeking treatment; such groups include women, the young, street children, refugees, the poor and minority ethnic and religious groups.

Collecting data on the number of patients treated with each type of treatment can be useful. Data on numbers in opioid agonist maintenance treatment can be gathered from treatment centres or pharmacies dispensing methadone and buprenorphine, either in real time or on an intermittent basis. Gathering data on numbers of people treated for opioid withdrawal is more difficult, and requires coordination of data from residential facilities, outpatient specialist services and primary care. A relatively inexpensive way to evaluate long-term outcomes is to link data records with population registries (mortality).

A needs assessment is a formal systematic attempt to determine important gaps between what services are needed and those that are currently being provided. The assessment involves documenting important gaps between current and desired outcomes, and then deciding in which order those gaps should be closed.

When planning and developing pharmacological treatment for people with opioid dependence, the scope of present and potential public health problems associated with opioid dependence and current treatment coverage should be considered.

> **Recommendation** *(Best Practice)*
> A strategy document should be produced outlining the government policy on the treatment of opioid dependence. The strategy should aim for adequate coverage, quality and safety of treatment.

4.4 Ethical issues

4.4.1 COMPULSORY AND COERCED TREATMENT

In line with the principle of autonomy, patients should be free to choose whether to participate in treatment, unless another ethical principle overrides this. The principle of autonomy may be overridden, for example, when a person is incapacitated by a mental illness and can no longer care for themselves, or when a person poses a risk to others. Most countries have mental health legislation to this effect, which can be applied to patients with opioid dependence if necessary. However, in most cases, those who have lost control over opioid use are not necessarily considered to have lost the ability to care for themselves in other ways.

In situations where opioid-dependent individuals are convicted of crimes related to their opioid use, they may be offered treatment for their opioid dependence as an alternative to a penal sanction. Such treatment would not be considered compulsory unless the punishment for refusing or failing treatment were more severe than the penal sanction it replaced. Similarly, legal proceedings can be a delayed until after a period of treatment, so that the effects of treatment can be taken into account. Such programmes, which divert opioid-dependent patients away from the criminal justice system, can also be implemented on arrest or before trial. These programmes are sometimes called diversion programmes (the use of the term "diversion" here should not be confused with its use in "diversion of treatment medication", which is described elsewhere). Evaluations of diversion programmes show high rates of successful treatment and low rates of recidivism[53, 54].

> **Recommendation** *(Minimum standard)*
> Psychosocially assisted pharmacological treatment should not be compulsory.

4.4.2 CENTRAL REGISTRATION OF PATIENTS

Patients should have the right to privacy. Confidentiality should be considered when contemplating setting up systems of central registration of patients. Central registration has advantages, in that it:
- prevents patients from receiving methadone or buprenorphine from more than one source
- can be used to limit access to other controlled medicines requiring central approval, such as other opioids
- can provide more accurate data on treatment numbers than situations where central registration is not used.

However, central registration can facilitate breaches of privacy, and this may deter some patients from entering treatment. It can also delay the commencement of treatment.

Safe and effective treatment of opioid dependence can be achieved without central registration. Because such registration could cause harm if privacy is breached, it should only be used if government agencies have effective systems for maintaining privacy.

4.5 Funding

In each national situation, funding and equitable access to treatment should be assured for the treatment approaches that are appropriate. In general, this means making the most cost-effective treatment widely available and accessible.

The cost to patients of treatment for opioid dependence also influences the outcomes of treatment. If costs are excessive, treatment will not be accessible to disadvantaged populations. Many opioid-dependent patients have difficulty paying for treatment and are not covered by health-insurance schemes. Where patients have to pay for treatment, retention rates and health outcomes are worse than where treatment is free[55]. Even small financial costs for treatment can be a significant disincentive.

Costing mechanisms for treatment can have unintended consequences. For example, if higher doses of methadone and buprenorphine cost more than lower doses, patients may opt for too low a dose, resulting in poorer outcomes. In contrast, if patients pay the same price regardless of the dose, they may overstate their needs and sell their excess supply, which in turn may make staff reluctant to increase the medication dose when patients request it.

The cost of dispensing the medication is also relevant. If patients pay a dispensing fee to a pharmacist or clinic each time they collect their medication, they may collect their medication less frequently.

Although it is impossible to avoid all perverse incentives (i.e. those that have unintended and undesirable effects), making treatment both free and accessible will minimize them.

Where a country has a public universal health-care system, this should include access to opioid dependence treatment. Where a country has an insurance system, this should again include access to opioid dependence treatment, recognizing that long-term treatment will be needed in many cases.

Another aspect of treatment funding is sustainability. In many cases, pilot funding is used to launch treatment of opioid dependence. However, it is not appropriate to use short-term funding for long-term agonist maintenance treatment without a realistic prospect of people in treatment being able to access continuing pharmacotherapy at the end of the pilot phase.

The development and maintenance of opioid treatment services evidently needs to take place within the broader system of health-care financing and provision in a given country. An understanding of the way that health funds are raised and allocated in a country is therefore important for the appropriate planning of opioid treatment services. One particularly important potential barrier to treatment in many countries with relatively low resources is the reliance on private, out-of-pocket spending by households as the primary mechanism for paying for health care. Tax-based public health-insurance schemes provide a more equitable mechanism for paying for health services, as well as a more suitable basis for developing and sustaining opioid treatment services at the population level.

Determining the total resources and associated costs needed to initiate and maintain a treatment service for opioid dependence should be a key element of strategic planning. Although cost estimates have been produced for a range of opioid-dependence treatment programmes [56, 57, 58, 59, 60, 61, 62, 63], they are largely restricted to the context of high-income countries, where costs and levels of funding for health may differ markedly from those found in low and middle-income countries. For example, although estimates of required staff will figure prominently in any resource-planning exercise, the costs of this labour may not represent such a large component of total cost in low and middle-income countries (due to lower salary levels); in contrast, the costs of purchasing and distributing medication, and of fuel, utilities and equipment may take up a relatively greater share of costs in such countries. WHO has methods and tools that can be used to assist such resource planning and programme costing at the national level[64].

> **Recommendation** *(Minimum standard)*
> Treatment should be accessible to disadvantaged populations.
>
> **Recommendation** *(Minimum standard)*
> At the time of commencement of treatment services, there should be a realistic prospect of the service being financially viable.
>
> **Recommendation** *(Best Practice)*
> To achieve optimal coverage and treatment outcomes, treatment of opioid dependence should be provided free of charge, or covered by public health-care insurance.

4.6 Coverage

Pharmacological treatment of opioid dependence should be accessible to all those in need, including those in prison (the efficacy of opioid agonist maintenance treatment is well documented in this setting) and other closed settings[65, 66, 67]. Interruptions to opioid agonist maintenance treatment while patients are moving in and out of custodial settings should be avoided.

Treatment programmes should be designed to be as accessible as possible; for example, programmes should be physically accessible, open at convenient times, have no undue restrictions on accessibility, and have the capacity to be expanded to accommodate likely demand. A programme should provide adequate facilities and should have opening hours that allow staff and patient confidentiality and safety, adequate and accessible dispensing facilities, and safe and secure storage of medications.

> **Recommendation** *(Minimum standard)*
> Pharmacological treatment of opioid dependence should be widely accessible; this might include treatment delivery in primary care settings. Comorbid patients can be treated in primary health-care settings if there is access to specialist consultation when necessary.
>
> **Recommendation** *(Best Practice)*
> Pharmacological treatment of opioid dependence should be accessible to all those in need, including those in prison and other closed settings.

4.6.1 PRIMARY CARE

Integration of opioid dependence treatment into primary care is one way to increase accessibility, although it may not be possible in all settings. Primary care practitioners will usually need support from the specialist system, through mentoring, training, consultation and referral. With such support, patients with quite complex comorbidity can be safely managed in primary care.

Opioid agonist maintenance treatment, opioid withdrawal services and relapse prevention services can all be provided in primary care settings, given the right conditions.

Several clinical trials of opioid agonist maintenance treatment have been conducted in primary care settings[68, 69, 70]. Use of general practitioners for opioid agonist maintenance treatment significantly increases the capacity of the service, and treatment numbers have increased rapidly in countries that have adopted this approach[71]. Treatment in primary care also has the advantage of integrating addiction medical and psychiatric services into mainstream services, reducing the stigma of addiction and the professional isolation of medical staff. Integration also reduces some of the problems that clinics can develop when large numbers of patients on opioid agonist maintenance are aggregated. Within the clinic setting, interaction between patients can lead to drug dealing and an antitherapeutic milieu. Outside the clinic, the congregation of drug users can become a visible target for members of the public who do not approve of opioid agonist maintenance treatment.

Opioid withdrawal and relapse prevention services can also be provided in primary care, with similar efficacy as specialist clinics but at lower cost[72, 73].

4.6.2 PRISONS

Prisoners should not be denied adequate health care because of their imprisonment. This would normally imply that the treatment options available outside prison should also be available in prison. Opioid withdrawal, agonist maintenance and naltrexone treatment should all be available in prison settings, and prisoners should not be forced to accept any particular treatment.

Opioid agonist treatment in prisons

The benefits of opioid agonist maintenance in prisons include less injecting drug use while in prison, increase in uptake of treatment on leaving prison, and reduction of rates of return to prison. Potential harms include diversion of medication, and spread of HIV through injection of diverted medication using contaminated injecting equipment. Because of these potential harms, unsupervised doses are generally not appropriate in prison settings. Rates of diversion of methadone are low, even in prison settings, and can be reduced further by diluting the methadone and by keeping methadone patients separate from other prisoners for 30 minutes after dosing.

Because it is a sublingual tablet that can take up to 15 minutes to dissolve, buprenorphine is difficult to supervise in prison settings, sometimes resulting in pressure on patients from other prisoners to divert their medication for injection[74]. Methods to increase the effectiveness of supervision include crushing the tablet, filming dosing, ensuring the hands remain behind the back of the patient during dosing and inspecting the mouth after dosing. If effective supervision of buprenorphine is difficult, it may be better to use methadone instead.

Policy makers and prison administrators should ensure appropriate links between prison health services and agonist maintenance treatment outside prison. Even small gaps in the continuity of treatment are distressing for the patient and risk the person relapsing to illicit opioid use. Therefore, opioid agonist maintenance treatment should be continuous on leaving prison. This means coordinating the day of discharge from prison with the day of commencement of opioid agonist treatment outside prison.

Patients not in treatment in prison should be given the opportunity to start methadone or buprenorphine in prison, even if they have only a short period of their sentence left to complete. Commencement of opioid agonist maintenance treatment in prison reduces the high risk of overdose and death on leaving prison, and reduces reincarceration rates.

4.7 What treatments should be available?

If countries are able to afford it, it is best to have both methadone and buprenorphine available for opioid agonist maintenance treatment. Having both treatments means that patients who experience adverse effects from one of the medications, or fail to respond, can try the alternative. This situation may increase the proportion of people with opioid dependence staying in opioid agonist treatment; it may also increase the effectiveness of treatment, through better matching of treatment and patient. The additional availability of alpha-2 adrenergic agonists for opioid withdrawal increases the options for those who wish to withdraw as quickly as possible or who wish to commence naltrexone after withdrawal. The availability of naltrexone after withdrawal is also a valuable additional option, because it gives a lower rate of relapse.

> **Recommendation** *(Minimum standard)*
> Essential pharmacological treatment options should consist of opioid agonist maintenance treatment and services for the management of opioid withdrawal. At a minimum, this would include either methadone or buprenorphine for opioid agonist maintenance and outpatient withdrawal management.
>
> **Recommendation** *(Best Practice)*
>
> Pharmacological treatment options should consist of both methadone and buprenorphine for opioid agonist maintenance and opioid withdrawal, alpha-2 adrenergic agonists for opioid withdrawal, naltrexone for relapse prevention , and naloxone for the treatment of overdose.

4.8 Supervision of dosing for methadone and buprenorphine maintenance

This section should be read with the section on opioid agonist maintenance treatment (Section 6.4). Without supervision of dosing, methadone and buprenorphine are likely to be diverted for illicit use, giving rise to problems of overdose, injection and spread of bloodborne viruses.

However, supervision of every dose is severely restrictive to patients, and limits the acceptability of treatment. Supervision of most doses is still onerous for patients, but is not necessarily detrimental to the individual in treatment; on the contrary, it may be of benefit in the early phases of treatment.

Regulations and laws describing the degree of supervision of methadone and buprenorphine maintenance should be in accordance with the relevant international treaties and reflect the balance between treatment acceptability and risk of diversion that is acceptable to the community. Programmes in which medicine is being diverted to the street market are not beneficial to patients and often not tolerated outside the health-care sector either. With guidance, treatment staff can select patients at lower risk of diversion, who can receive a lower level of supervision of dosing (Section 4.6).

In most cases, staff training, adequate take-home policies and normal legal restrictions on illicitly procured opioids can minimize diversion without the need for specific legislation. Programmes will be more sustainable if there are systems to prevent or minimize diversion of pharmacotherapy, and to monitor the benefits of treatment. As a minimum, this would include systems that monitor the extent of diversion (Section 5.7).

5 Programme level guidelines – for programme managers and clinical leaders

This section is primarily aimed at clinical leaders and health administrators responsible for the organization and delivery of opioid dependence treatment, and the standards of care involved.

5.1 Clinical governance

Clinical governance refers to the mechanism of accountability for clinical outcomes. Normally, this role falls to a clinical leader or health administrator, or is shared by both. Responsibilities include ensuring that:
- staff are adequately selected, trained and supervised
- adequate clinical protocols and procedures are in place for
  - determining the structure of the treatment service
  - developing and maintaining mechanisms of quality assessment and improvement
  - ensuring that practices comply with relevant laws and professional requirements.

As a minimum, a process of clinical governance should be established to ensure that minimal standards for provision of opioid dependence treatment are being met. Ideally, the process of clinical governance should be well developed, so that treatments for opioid dependence are both safe and effective.

Where treatment is delivered outside the health-care system (e.g. in prisons) and not primarily under the responsibility of health authorities, there should still be a documented chain of accountability for health outcomes.

It is best to have the primary responsibility for treatment within the health-care system, even in diverse settings, because clinical accountability is then easier to establish and maintain.

> **Recommendation** *(Minimum standard)*
> Treatment services should have a system of clinical governance, with a chain of clinical accountability within the health-care system, to ensure that the minimal standards for provision of opioid dependence treatment are being met.
>
> **Recommendation** *(Best Practice)*
> Treatment of opioid dependence should be provided within the health-care system.

> **Recommendation** *(Best Practice)*
> A process of clinical governance should be established to ensure that treatments for opioid dependence are both safe and effective. The process should be transparent and outlined in a clinical governance document.

5.2 Ethical principles and consent

In line with the rights to autonomy and the highest attainable standard of health enshrined in Article 12 of the International Covenant on Economic, Social and Cultural Rights[75], people should be free to chose whether or not they participate in treatment.

The *WHO Resource Book on Mental Health, Human Rights and Legislation*[76] says that, to be valid, consent must satisfy the following criteria:
- "The person/patient giving consent must be competent to do so, and competence is assumed unless there is evidence to the contrary.
- Consent must be obtained freely, without threats or improper inducements.
- There should be appropriate and adequate disclosure of information. Information must be provided on the purpose, method, likely duration and expected benefits of the proposed treatment; possible pain or discomfort and risks of the proposed treatment, and likely side-effects. This information should be adequately discussed with the patient.
- Choices should be offered, if available, in accordance with good clinical practice; alternative modes of treatment, especially those that are less intrusive, should be discussed and offered to the patient.
- Information should be provided in a language and form that is understandable to the patient.
- The patient should have the right to refuse or stop treatment.
- Consequences of refusing treatment, which may include discharge from the hospital, should be explained to the patient.
- The consent should be documented in the patient's medical records.
- The right to consent to treatment implies also the right to refuse treatment. If a patient is judged as

having the capacity to give consent, then refusal of such consent must also be respected."

One of the implications for provision of informed consent in opioid-dependent patients is that patients may not be in an adequate state to provide informed consent when they are intoxicated or in opioid withdrawal. In this case, treatment may commence and patients may be asked to confirm their consent to treatment after treatment has commenced, as soon as the patient is neither intoxicated nor in opioid withdrawal. On occasion, this may mean a change in treatment direction from opioid agonist maintenance to opioid withdrawal, or the reverse.

When considering what risks to include in the informed consent process for patients commencing opioid agonist maintenance treatment, it is important to include the increased risk of overdose during the first weeks of treatment, and the likely opioid withdrawal symptoms that will be experienced when stopping opioid agonist treatment. Patients commencing opioid withdrawal and abstinence-based treatments should be specifically warned about the increased risk of overdose on relapse to opioid use compared to opioid agonist maintenance treatment.

> **Recommendation** *(Minimum standard)*
> Patients must give informed consent for treatment.

5.3 Staff and training

The support and training of health-care personnel requires a continuous effort, and special attention is needed to develop and maintain a competent workforce. Training should include (as a minimum) an understanding of the nature of opioid dependence, assessment and diagnosis, pharmacological and psychosocial treatments, and management of intoxication, overdose and difficult behaviours.

> **Recommendation** *(Minimum standard)*
> Treatment of opioid dependence should be carried out by trained health-care personnel. The level of training for specific tasks should be determined by the level of responsibility and national regulations.

> **Recommendation** *(Best Practice)*
> Health authorities should ensure that treatment providers have sufficient skill and qualifications to use controlled substances appropriately. These requirements may include postgraduate training and certification, continuing education and licensing and the setting aside of funding for monitoring and evaluation.

5.3.1 MEDICAL STAFF

In most settings, medical staff will be required for the treatment of opioid dependence, both for clinical assessment and for prescription of pharmacotherapy. In some settings, due to a shortage of medical staff, these responsibilities may fall on nursing or other health-care staff. Also, medical staff may delegate some of their responsibilities to nursing and other health-care staff, in accordance with local regulations.

In specialist clinics, medical staff should be supervised by a physician or psychiatrist specializing in the treatment of substance dependence.

In generalist settings, general practitioners and other medical staff should have a basic level of training in the diagnosis and treatment of opioid dependence. Because of the potential for methadone and buprenorphine to do harm if prescribed inappropriately, many countries have a system of licensing medical staff to prescribe opioid agonist maintenance treatment. Each service should ensure that its own training programmes incorporate local clinical guidelines and regulations.

All medical staff working in the field of substance abuse should have some avenue for clinical supervision, be it from peers, senior colleagues or professional supervisors. This helps to guard against inappropriate prescribing and to maintain the professionalism of medical staff in their dealings with patients.

5.3.2 PHARMACY STAFF

Staff dispensing methadone and buprenorphine are generally pharmacists, although medical and nursing staff may also be able to dispense medication, depending on national laws. Staff dispensing methadone and buprenorphine should have specific training in opioid-dependence treatment. This should include the nature of opioid dependence, the goals of treatment, therapeutic rapport, recognition of opioid withdrawal and intoxication, and responses to difficult behaviours. This should include proper storage of controlled medicines, the nature of opioid dependence, the goals of treatment, therapeutic rapport, recognition of opioid withdrawal and intoxication, methods to minimize diversion of medication, and responses to difficult behaviours.

5.3.3 PSYCHOSOCIAL SUPPORT STAFF

To ensure professionalism and consistency of service delivery, basic training in treatment of substance dependence is recommended. Further training requirements will depend on the nature of the psychosocial intervention being offered.

Staff should be provided with supervision, adequate support, and standardized operational instructions on the management of intoxication, difficult behaviours and other emergency conditions.

5.4 Clinical records

Every contact between the health service and the patient should be recorded in the medical record. The record should be up to date and clearly legible. Each entry should be signed and dated.

Sometimes police may ask to see medical records; they should not be given access to medical records against the wishes of the patient unless appropriate legal requirements and procedures have been met.

In some circumstances, professional standards may warrant a breach of confidentiality; for example, if the safety of a child is at risk. In these situations, professional staff should balance the patient's right to privacy against the duty to protect, and should seek advice from their professional body if unsure. Such breaches of confidentiality are generally allowed under law; indeed, in some cases they may be required by law.

As a general rule, patients should have access to their own medical records. This may be limited in some situations if it is not in the patient's best interest to view all of his or her own records.

If there are national systems of identification, such as identity cards, bank cards or social security cards, these should be used when necessary to confirm the identity of patients. In the absence of such systems, treatment providers should find alternative ways to establish patient identity. The main reason for this is to avoid giving potentially lethal doses of opioids to the wrong patient. If there is a system of central registration (Section 4.2), the system will require accurate identification of participants if it is to be effective.

> **Recommendation** *(Minimum standard)*
> Up-to-date medical records should be kept for all patients. These should include, as a minimum, the history, clinical examination, investigations, diagnosis, health and social status, treatment plans and their revisions, referrals, evidence of consent, prescribed drugs and other interventions received.
>
> **Recommendation** *(Minimum standard)*
> Confidentiality of patient records should be ensured.
>
> **Recommendation** *(Minimum standard)*
> Health-care providers involved in the treatment of an individual should have access to patient data in accordance with national regulations, as should patients themselves.
>
> **Recommendation** *(Minimum standard)*
> Health-care providers or other personnel involved in patient treatment should not share information about patients with police and other law enforcement authorities unless a patient approves, or unless required by law.
>
> **Recommendation** *(Minimum standard)*
> Patients treated with opioid agonists should be identifiable to treating staff.

5.5 Medication safety

Most countries have regulations that govern the procurement, storage, dispensing and dosing of medicines, and these often contain special provisions for opioids and other medications of abuse and dependence. The regulations usually stipulate storage of methadone and buprenorphine in locked cabinets, with two staff members witnessing any movement of medication. These measures reduce the risk of theft of medication, particularly the risk of diversion by staff members.

Methadone and buprenorphine can be fatal if the wrong dose is dispensed or a dose is dispensed to the wrong patient. Various systems can be used to ensure that the correct dose is being dispensed to the correct patient. Such systems essentially involve checking the identity of the patient and ensuring that the prescription is valid. They can be low technology – for example, having a photo of the patient at the dispensing point and having the patient sign for their dose. Alternatively, systems can be high-technology – for example, commercial systems linking retinal scanning devices to methadone pumps.

> **Recommendation** *(Minimum standard)*
> Documented processes should be established to ensure the safe and legal procurement, storage, dispensing and dosing of medicines, particularly of methadone and buprenorphine.

5.6 Treatment provision

5.6.1 CLINICAL GUIDELINES

Clinical guidelines are one mechanism for improving the quality of treatment. Clear, evidence-based clinical guidelines for the treatment of opioid dependence are available, and at a minimum these should be accessible to treatment staff. Ideally, local guidelines should be developed at a country or subnational level to reflect local laws, policies and conditions. The guidelines will be affected by differences in costs and requirements for supervision of methadone and buprenorphine. Local guidelines should represent the accepted treatment standards in the particular location, reflecting to some extent the values and mores of the society and its professional bodies.

> **Recommendation** *(Minimum standard)*
> Clinical guidelines for the treatment of opioid dependence should be available to clinical staff.
>
> **Recommendation** *(Best Practice)*
> Clinical guidelines should be detailed, comprehensive, evidence based and developed at a country level or lower, to reflect local laws, policies and conditions.

5.6.2 TREATMENT POLICIES

Policies on the objectives, indications, settings, dosage schemes and treatment regulations (including reasons for treatment termination) should be developed and clearly communicated to patients and staff. This applies for the management of opioid dependence with opioid detoxification, opioid agonist maintenance and naltrexone treatment.

Access to and networking with medical, psychiatric, social and harm-reduction services is desirable, and should be developed when possible; however, psychosocial interventions, including counselling, may not be necessary onsite.

Men and women can be treated in the same facility, providing that culturally appropriate and gender-specific needs can be taken care of.

> **Recommendation** *(Minimum standard)*
> To maximize the safety and effectiveness of agonist maintenance treatment programmes, policies and regulations should encourage flexible dosing structures, with low starting doses and high maintenance doses, without placing restrictions on dose levels and the duration of treatment.
>
> **Recommendation** *(Best Practice)*
> Opioid withdrawal services should be structured such that withdrawal is not a stand-alone service but is integrated with ongoing treatment options.
>
> **Recommendation** *(Best Practice)*
> Take-home doses can be recommended when the dose and social situation are stable, and when there is a low risk of diversion for illegitimate purposes.
>
> **Recommendation** *(Best Practice)*
> Involuntary discharge from treatment is justified to ensure the safety of staff and other patients, but noncompliance with programme rules alone should not generally be a reason for involuntary discharge. Before involuntary discharge, reasonable measures to improve the situation should be taken, including re-evaluation of the treatment approach used.

5.6.3 INVOLUNTARY DISCHARGE AND OTHER FORMS OF LIMIT SETTING

One of the primary responsibilities of a treatment

service is to protect its staff and patients from harm. If a situation arises in which the past behaviour of a patient would indicate that there is a significant risk of harm to other patients or staff, the treatment service must act to reduce that risk, discharging the patient if necessary. Such situations are potentially avoidable if the patient's behaviour is identified and managed at an early stage. An effective treatment service will have clear boundaries on what constitutes acceptable and unacceptable behaviour, and the service will apply the limits consistently and transparently to all patients (sometimes referred to as "limit setting"). To avoid replicating the rejection that patients experience from other parts of society, limit setting should have a graded response, including:
- positive feedback for "good" behaviour
- measured responses for mild breaches of acceptable behaviour (e.g. warnings, fewer take-home dose privileges, more frequent medical visits, refusing or delaying doses if intoxicated)
- final responses (e.g. treatment discharge and, if necessary, calling the police) for serious breaches of acceptable behaviour.

Applying excessive responses for minor breaches of rules will result in many people being discharged when they could have gone on to do well from treatment. At the same time, failure to respond to significant breaches of rules risks harm to other patients and staff, and will not help the patient in question.

Each service will have to decide on its own rules and limits; these will depend on cultural norms, the goals of treatment in that setting and the policy environment that allows the treatment to continue. Treatment rules are likely to be very different for a withdrawal facility or therapeutic community aimed at abstinence, and an opioid agonist maintenance programme aimed at reducing the mortality and morbidity associated with opioid dependence, and at improving quality of life.

Whatever limits are set, they must be consistently applied by all treatment staff. In this way, patients will quickly learn and more readily accept the boundaries of acceptable behaviour. Some patients will push these boundaries when there is a perceived difference in the way that staff apply limits. Sometimes called "splitting", this behaviour risks setting treatment staff against each other, leading to poor outcomes for patients.

Even if an incident is sufficiently serious to warrant abrupt discharge, agencies should use this as an occasion to review whether they have done all they can to avoid provoking or permitting such behaviour. Treatment services should have a mechanism of reporting incidents when they occur, including "near misses" and unexpected adverse outcomes. The reports should be reviewed regularly by a team that includes someone responsible for the clinical governance of the service.

Initiatives to reduce such incidents might include measures to train staff in non-judgemental and non-confrontational communication strategies, reducing waiting time for appointments and medication, frequent review of patient treatment, use of family and employment-friendly practices, and presence of security.

If the situation does not warrant immediate discharge for the safety of staff and other patients, then attempts should be made to resolve the situation without discharge, particularly if discharge implies no continuing treatment. Patients should understand what is expected of them, and there should be clear communication when behaviour crosses the boundaries. When alternative options are inappropriate or have been exhausted, attempts should be made to transfer the patient to another treatment service, because outcomes after involuntary discharge from treatment are poor, with relapse to heroin use occurring in 75% of patients[77].

5.6.4 INDIVIDUAL TREATMENT PLANS

The first stage in individualized treatment is a thorough individual assessment that identifies specific psychosocial needs and patient motivations, and confirms the diagnosis of opioid dependence and the response to previous treatments (Section 6.1). Holistic treatment then attempts to meet each of those treatment needs. Where possible, interventions to address particular needs should be evidence based, incorporating individual preferences and past treatment experiences.

As with other long-term conditions, patients should not be assumed to be "cured" with the first round of treatment, and provisions should be made for follow-up. Treatment programmes should be structured in such a way that they can support patients in the long term.

> **Recommendation** *(Minimum standard)*
> A detailed individual assessment should be conducted which includes: history (past treatment experiences; medical and psychiatric history; living conditions; legal issues; occupational situation; and social and cultural factors, that may influence substance use); clinical examination (assessment of intoxication / withdrawal, injection marks); and, if necessary, investigations (such as urine drug screen, HIV, Hep C, Hep B, TB, liver function).
>
> **Recommendation** *(Best Practice)*
> Screening for psychiatric and somatic comorbidity should form part of the initial assessment.
>
> **Recommendation** *(Best Practice)*
> The choice of treatment for an individual should be based on a detailed assessment of the treatment needs, appropriateness of treatment to meet those needs (assessment of appropriateness should be evidence based), patient acceptance and treatment availability.
>
> **Recommendation** *(Best Practice)*
> Treatment plans should take a long-term perspective.
>
> **Recommendation** *(Best Practice)*
> Opioid detoxification should be planned in conjunction with ongoing treatment.

5.6.5 RANGE OF SERVICES TO BE PROVIDED

Although different treatment options may be available in different programmes, it is useful for programmes to be able to offer a full range of services, so that they can tailor the services to the needs of the patients.

Each treatment facility with medical staff should ensure that the facility has the capacity to administer the opioid antagonist naloxone to treat opioid overdoses. This includes procedures for maintaining stock and injection equipment. Distribution of naloxone, with training on its use in overdose to opioid users and their families, has been shown to be a feasible approach to reducing overdose mortality in the community[78, 79, 80]. It is similar in concept to the distribution of adrenaline to patients with severe allergic reactions and their families.

> **Recommendation** *(Minimum standard)*
> Essential pharmacological treatment options should consist of opioid agonist maintenance treatment and services for the management of opioid withdrawal.
>
> **Recommendation** *(Minimum standard)*
> Naloxone should be available for treating opioid overdose.
>
> **Recommendation** *(Best Practice)*
> Pharmacological treatment options should consist of both methadone and buprenorphine for opioid agonist maintenance and opioid withdrawal, alpha-2 adrenergic agonists for opioid withdrawal, naltrexone for relapse prevention, and naloxone for the treatment of overdose.

5.6.6 TREATMENT OF COMORBID CONDITIONS

Opioid-dependent patients often also suffer from other medical and psychiatric conditions, complicated by social problems. The optimal approach is to provide integrated holistic care to address current problems and prevent further problems. In practice, this means being able to detect medical, psychiatric and social issues in the assessment process, and having the means onsite to attend to the issues simultaneously. This may mean having staff with multiple skills, or coordinating the use of staff with different skill sets.

5.6.7 PSYCHOSOCIAL AND PSYCHIATRIC SUPPORT

Medications are useful in the treatment of opioid dependence. However, providing medications without offering any psychosocial assistance fails to recognize the complex nature of opioid dependence, loses the opportunity to provide optimal interventions and requires treatment staff to go against their clinical inclination to respond to the total needs of their patients. Treatment services should aim to offer onsite, integrated, comprehensive psychosocial support to every patient. However, treatment services should not deny effective medication if they are unable to provide psychosocial assistance, or if patients refuse it. At a minimum, services should attempt to assess the psychosocial needs of patients, provide whatever support they can, and refer to outside agencies for additional support where necessary.

> **Recommendation** *(Minimum standard)*
> Psychosocial support should be available to all opioid-dependent patients, in association with pharmacological treatments of opioid dependence. At a minimum, this should include assessment of psychosocial needs, supportive counselling and links to existing family and community services.
>
> **Recommendation** *(Best Practice)*
> A variety of structured psychosocial interventions should be available, according to the needs of the patients. Such interventions may include - but are not limited to - different forms of counselling and psychotherapy, and assistance with social needs such as housing, employment, education, welfare and legal problems.
>
> **Recommendation** *(Best Practice)*
> Onsite psychosocial and psychiatric treatment should be provided for patients with psychiatric comorbidity.

5.6.8 TB, HEPATITIS AND HIV

Despite the large number of opioid-dependent people living with HIV/AIDS, there is considerable evidence that they have less access to antiretroviral medication, and to other HIV/AIDS treatment and care than others who are not substance dependent. Opioid use has been identified as a factor in lack of adherence to antiretroviral treatment, risking the development of viral drug resistance[81].

On the other hand, observational studies suggest that the impact of highly active antiretroviral therapy on CD4 counts in patients still using heroin and other drugs is reasonable, and is not too dissimilar to the impact of such therapy in patients not using illicit substances[82]. Excellent results can be obtained for patients in opioid agonist maintenance treatment[83].

The issues for TB and hepatitis treatment are similar, with the exception that clinics with TB patients need to carefully consider the risks of spread of TB from patient to patient, particularly where immunocompromised patients are mixing with TB patients. Given the capacity for overcrowded clinics to spread TB, opioid-dependence treatment clinics should consider their response to the issue of TB in combination with local TB experts. Issues of ventilation, overcrowding and management of coughing patients may need to be considered.

Combined treatment of hepatitis C and opioid dependence with opioid agonist maintenance treatment and anti-viral agents can also have excellent results[84, 85, 86, 87].

A number of RCTs have demonstrated that substance-dependent patients are more likely to attend for medical care if the treatment is provided onsite; this can be arranged for minimal additional cost[88, 89, 90, 91, 92, 93]. An alternative approach – providing opioid agonist maintenance treatment at medical clinics[94] – has also been suggested.

To improve compliance, directly observed treatment of HIV and TB should be integrated with opioid agonist maintenance treatment, and provided in the same location.

There are a number of models for the development of such integrated care.
- Existing opioid-dependence programmes may start treating medical conditions[84].
- Existing medical programmes may start treating opioid dependence[85].
- New specialized services for drug users may treat opioid dependence, TB, HIV and hepatitis.
- Opioid dependence and HIV/TB can be treated in primary care[87].

According to local conditions, mechanisms for treating opioid dependence should be combined with treatment for TB, HIV and hepatitis. The simplest way for this to happen may be for treatment staff to become skilled in treating multiple conditions. Since patients on opioid agonist maintenance treatment already attend a clinic or dispensary daily, integration with HIV treatment provides an efficient mechanism for directly observing HIV treatment and achieving high compliance rates. Where there is no capacity to provide integrated care, links should be established between services providing drug treatment and services providing treatment for HIV, TB and hepatitis, to increase the success of referral and treatment.

Patients with active TB are highly infective and should be kept separate from other patients as much as possible in the initial stages of treatment, particularly during the first two weeks of anti-TB therapy.

All injecting drug users should have access to measures to reduce the spread of HIV, including access to clean injecting equipment, condoms, antiretroviral drugs and other treatments, psychosocial services and medical care. While patients who have ceased heroin use before treatment have higher rates of adherence to antiretroviral treatment, patients without a drug-free period also have acceptable levels of response to treatment, and there should be no absolute requirement for patients to be drug free before commencing treatment.

> **Recommendation** (Minimum standard)
> Links to HIV, hepatitis and TB treatment services (where they exist) should be provided.
>
> **Recommendation** (Best Practice)
> Where there are significant numbers of opioid-dependent patients in need of treatment for either HIV, hepatitis or TB, treatment of opioid dependence should be integrated with medical services for these conditions.
>
> **Recommendation** (Best Practice)
> For opioid-dependent patients with TB, hepatitis or HIV, opioid agonists should be administered in conjunction with other medical treatment; there is no need to wait for abstinence from opioids to commence either anti-TB medication, treatment for hepatitis or antiretroviral medication.
>
> **Recommendation** (Best Practice)
> Opioid-dependent patients with TB, hepatitis or HIV should have equitable access to treatment for TB, hepatitis, HIV and opioid dependence.

5.6.9 HEPATITIS B VACCINATION

Vaccination for hepatitis B is recommended for all opioid-dependent patients[95]. Ideally, hepatitis B vaccines should be given in three doses at least four weeks apart, but other vaccination schedules can also provide acceptable protection. Each treatment service should establish its own vaccination policy, based on the costs of vaccination and serology testing, the ability to maintain a cold chain, the prevalence of hepatitis B and the likelihood that patients will come back for follow-up appointments. Given the difficulty of bringing patients back for follow-up appointments and the relatively low cost of the *Vaccine*. vaccinating all patients without prior serology testing may be the most effective and the most cost-effective approach, even if completion of the course is not guaranteed. Some studies have shown that provision of free *Vaccine*. staff training, incentives, onsite vaccination and accelerated schedules can result in higher vaccination rates in this population[96, 97, 98]

On the other hand, it is useful to test levels of post-vaccination anti-hepatitis B antibodies, because significant numbers of people do not produce an adequate immune response[99, 100, 101]; in these cases, additional doses of vaccination should be given.

Many opioid-dependent patients will also benefit from vaccination against hepatitis A[102].

> **Recommendation** (Best Practice)
> Treatment services should offer hepatitis B vaccination to all opioid-dependent patients.

5.7 Treatment evaluation

For opioid agonist maintenance treatment programmes, monitoring the potential for harm through diversion, overdose and other adverse events should be the minimum standard of treatment evaluation. Examples of simple evaluation techniques that could be used to detect diversion of drugs from treatment include interviewing key informants about drug diversion and testing levels of the main drugs used in patients presenting for treatment.

A system of detecting and recording adverse events in treatment, followed by regular discussion and implementation of necessary changes, will help to ensure safety. Following-up patients who drop out of treatment is helpful in this regard.

Optimal treatment evaluation examines safety, effectiveness and processes of care. Effectiveness can be measured "in house", through routine collection of outcome measures combined with follow-up of those who have left the service, or "externally", with the assistance of an external evaluation person or team.

Further details on evaluation can be found in the WHO toolkit on the evaluation of opioid substitution programmes[103].

Recommendation (Minimum standard)
There should be a system for monitoring the safety of the treatment service, including the extent of medication diversion.

Recommendation (Best Practice)
There should be intermittent or ongoing evaluation of both the process and the outcomes of the treatment provided.

6 Patient level guidelines – for clinicians

In recent years, the choice of treatment options for opioid dependence has expanded. Although opioid agonist maintenance treatments (methadone and buprenorphine) are increasingly seen as the most effective management strategies, other options are opioid withdrawal and relapse prevention. In practice, different approaches will suit different patients. Many patients will undergo several episodes of different forms of treatment before finding treatments that work for them. The choice between the treatment options available should be made jointly by the clinician and patient, taking into account the priorities of the patient, the principles of medical ethics and the evidence for effectiveness of the treatments, as well as individual patient factors, such as past treatment history.

The three treatment approaches discussed in this section are:
- opioid agonist maintenance treatment
- opioid withdrawal
- opioid withdrawal followed by oral naltrexone.

The issues considered in relation to opioid agonist maintenance treatment are:
- methadone compared to buprenorphine for maintenance treatment
- optimal doses of methadone and buprenorphine
- use of adjuvant psychosocial support.

The issues considered in relation to opioid withdrawal are:
- choice of medication - methadone, buprenorphine or alpha-2 adrenergic agonists (e.g. clonidine and lofexidine)
- use of accelerated opioid withdrawal techniques with opioid antagonists (e.g. naloxone and naltrexone) with either minimal or heavy sedation
- use of oral naltrexone for relapse prevention after opioid withdrawal
- use of psychosocial support as an adjuvant to the above therapies
- choice between inpatient and outpatient detoxification services.

6.1 Diagnosis and assessment of opioid dependence

Assessment includes establishing a relationship between the patient and the treatment staff, based on the free exchange of information. Initially, patients may wish to share only information required to start the treatment process. However, as trust develops between the patient and staff, more information may be shared, and treatment staff will be better able to tailor responses to the individual patient.

Determining the physical, psychological and social health-care needs of the patient is an important part of assessment. Assessment should also include factors that may influence drug use, such as past treatment experiences, living conditions, legal issues, occupational situation, and social and cultural factors.

The clinician should take a substance use history to assess:
- which psychoactive substances have been used in the past, and which are currently being used
- the pattern of use for each substance, including information on the quantity and frequency of use
- the current level of neuroadaptation to each substance used
- drug induced health and social problems
- previous responses to treatment and other interventions
- whether the criteria for harmful use or dependence are met
- how the patient views their substance use
- the factors that have contributed, and continue to contribute, to the patient's use of psychoactive substances
- the short, medium and long-term goals of the patient, and what has brought the patient to the treatment facility on this occasion.

Clinicians should differentiate between substance dependence and nondependent harmful substance use, because these categories have significant implications for the appropriate treatment strategy.

On examination of the patient, the degree of intoxication or withdrawal should be interpreted in combination with the stated time of last use.[1] If there is a history of injection, the injection sites should be visible and consistent with the stated history (usually both recent and old injection marks will be visible).

6.1.1 URINE DRUG SCREENING

Where available and affordable, urine (or other biological sample) drug screening should be routinely conducted at the start of treatment, and should indicate recent opioid use if the person is to be eligible for treatment. When the cost of urine testing is an issue, urine testing should be used at least when a recent history of opioid use cannot be verified by other means (e.g. evidence of opioid withdrawal or intoxication). A negative urine drug screen combined with absence of withdrawal symptoms excludes current neuroadaptation to opioids; however, it does not exclude dependence on opioids in the past 12 months. Thus, dependence should not be diagnosed on urine drug screening alone, but a negative urine drug screen in the absence withdrawal symptoms should prompt caution in the use of opioids and other sedative medication.

Urine testing is also useful, in combination with the history, to identify other substances that have recently been consumed.

Entry into appropriate treatment programmes should not be delayed by waiting for the result of urine drug screening, unless the other findings in the assessment raise concern about the diagnosis.

Naloxone challenge testing should not be used routinely to confirm the presence of current neuroadaptation, because it can induce significant withdrawal effects. The same information can normally be gathered from the patient's history, examination of the person and interpretation of urine drug test results. Provided the patient is informed of the risk of adverse effects, naloxone challenge testing can be used as an alternative to urine drug screening, to confirm the absence of current neuroadaptation (e.g. when considering giving an opioid antagonist to start maintenance treatment). In this situation, an accidental positive reaction is likely to be significantly milder than the reaction that occurs when the test is used to confirm current neuroadaptation.

6.1.2 TESTING FOR INFECTIOUS DISEASES

Voluntary testing for HIV, hepatitis C and common infectious diseases should be offered as part of an individual assessment, accompanied by counselling before and after the test. In areas of high prevalence of HIV, patients should be strongly encouraged to undergo HIV testing. Serology testing and vaccination for hepatitis B is also recommended. As discussed above (Section 5.6), in some circumstances it may be more effective to vaccinate before testing for hepatitis B, and to use accelerated vaccination schedules.

TB and sexually transmitted diseases should also be considered during assessment.

Pregnancy testing should be offered to all women, particularly those contemplating opioid withdrawal, because it may influence the choice of treatment.

6.1.3 IDENTIFYING THE PATIENT

In some circumstances, it may be necessary to confirm the identity of the patient, particularly if treatment with controlled medicines is anticipated. Where patients do not have formal identification, it is advisable to take a photograph and include it in the record signed by the treating clinician, so that the patient can be identified in that clinic. The identity of the patient should be kept private and should not be released without patient consent. When collecting and recording information, the capacity of the service to keep that information private should be discussed with the patient.

6.1.4 COMPLETING THE ASSESSMENT

Sometimes it is not possible to complete the initial assessment in one day; for example, the patient may be intoxicated, in withdrawal or in crisis. In such cases, it may be necessary to make a plan based on the initial assessment, which will then evolve in response to a more

---

1 For example, see http://www.ncbi.nlm.nih.gov/books/bv.fcgi?rid=hstat5.chapter.72248

comprehensive assessment and the person's response to initial treatment.

6.1.4 DIAGNOSTIC CRITERIA

A diagnosis of opioid dependence has important prognostic and treatment implications. Once opioid dependent, the patient has a significant risk of suffering serious health consequences or of dying from behaviours related to their dependence on opioids.

The *International Classification of Diseases*, 10th edition (ICD-10) defines opioid dependence as "a cluster of physiological, behavioural, and cognitive phenomena in which the use of opioids takes on a much higher priority for a given individual than other behaviours that once had greater value". A central characteristic of the dependence syndrome is the desire (often strong, sometimes overpowering) to take opioids, which may or may not have been medically prescribed. Once a person is opioid dependent, returning to substance use after a period of abstinence leads to a more rapid reappearance of other features of the syndrome than occurs with nondependent individuals[104].

The ICD-10 diagnostic criteria for opioid dependence are:
- a strong desire or sense of compulsion to take opioids
- difficulties in controlling opioid-use behaviours in terms of the onset, termination or levels of use
- a physiological withdrawal state when opioid use has ceased or been reduced, as evidenced by one of the following
  - the characteristic withdrawal syndrome
  - use of opioids (or closely related substances) with the intention of relieving or avoiding withdrawal symptoms
- evidence of tolerance, such that increased doses of opioids are required to achieve effects originally produced by lower doses
- progressive neglect of alternative pleasures or interests because of opioid use
- increased amounts of time spent on obtaining opioids or recovering from their effects
- persisting with opioid use despite clear evidence of overtly harmful consequences, such as depressive mood states consequent to periods of heavy substance use, or drug-related impairment of cognitive functioning (efforts should be made to determine whether the user was actually, or could be expected to be, aware of the nature and extent of the harm).

Narrowing of the personal repertoire of patterns of opioid use has also been described as a characteristic feature of dependence.

Opioid dependence does not develop without a period of regular use, although regular use alone is not sufficient to induce dependence.

A definite diagnosis of dependence should usually be made only if three or more of the diagnostic criteria have been experienced or exhibited at some time during the previous year.

6.1.5 MAKING THE DIAGNOSIS

Opioid dependence is essentially diagnosed on the basis of the history provided by the patient. Patients can sometimes be motivated to either overstate or understate their substance use; therefore, it is usually necessary to corroborate the patient history with the results of the physical examination and investigations, and sometime with the history reported by significant others, to be confident of the diagnosis. While any health-care worker can make a provisional diagnosis of opioid dependence provided that they have had appropriate training, the diagnosis should be confirmed by medical staff before opioid agonist treatment is provided.

Injection sites

Examination of injection sites can provide useful information on the timing and duration of injecting drug use. Recent injection marks are small and red, and are sometimes inflamed or surrounded by slight bruising. Old injection sites are generally not inflamed, but sometimes show pigmentation changes (either lighter or darker), and the skin may have atrophied, giving a sunken impression. A combination of recent and old injection sites would normally be seen in an opioid-dependent patient with current neuroadaptation. Many sites can be used for injection, although the cubital fossa (the area on the inside of the elbow joint) and the groin are the most common.

Interpretation of urine drug screens

Urine drug screens provide evidence of recent drug use; this information can contribute to the assessment. The precise interpretation of a test result will depend on the specific commercial test or reagents used. Generally speaking, a positive test for the opioid class of drugs indicates the use of illicit or prescription opioids in the last few days. However, positive reactions can also be caused by large amounts of poppy seeds. Many commercial opioid drug screens do not recognise buprenorphine, but this situation is changing; therefore, it is best to check with the laboratory. Some tests, such as gas-chromatography and mass spectrometry (GCMS), can determine the specific opioid. Heroin is broken down to 6-monoacetylmorphine (6-MAM), then to morphine and then to codeine; thus, the presence of 6-MAM is usually specific for heroin use in the last 24 hours. Morphine, with or without small amounts of codeine, can indicate either heroin or morphine use in the last few days. Small amounts of morphine in the presence of large amounts of codeine can suggest intake of high doses of codeine, since codeine can also be metabolized to morphine although most is metabolized via a different pathway.

Degree of opioid intoxication and withdrawal

Features of opioid intoxication include drooping eyelids and constricted pupils, sedation, reduced respiratory rate, head nodding, and itching and scratching (due to histamine release).

Features of opioid withdrawal include yawning, anxiety, muscle aches, abdominal cramps, headache, dilated pupils, difficulty sleeping, vomiting, diarrhoea, piloerection (gooseflesh), agitation, myoclonic jerks, restlessness, delirium, seizures and elevated respiratory rate, blood pressure and pulse. Annex 10 provides useful scales for assessing the severity of opioid withdrawal.

6.2 Choice of treatment approach

Should agonist maintenance therapy (i.e. methadone or buprenorphine maintenance) be used in preference to withdrawal and oral antagonist therapy (naltrexone) or withdrawal alone?

> See evidence profiles in Annex 1 in:
> Sections A1.1 and A1.2 for methadone versus withdrawal
> Section A1.3 for buprenorphine versus withdrawal or placebo
> Section A1.11 for naltrexone versus placebo.

Efficacy

Methadone versus withdrawal

The recently updated Cochrane review[105] of methadone maintenance therapy versus no opioid replacement therapy identified three randomized controlled trials (RCTs) that compared methadone with opioid withdrawal followed by placebo[106, 107, 108]. These studies show that, compared to opioid withdrawal or placebo, methadone maintenance treatment dramatically reduces levels of illicit opioid use (relative risk [RR] 0.32; 95% confidence interval [CI] 0.23 to 0.44, high quality evidence) and increases retention in treatment (RR 3.05; 95%CI 1.75 to 5.35). Observational studies demonstrate that the mortality rate in methadone treatment is approximately one third the rate out of treatment (RR 0.37; 95%CI 0.29 to 0.48, low-quality evidence).

Methadone appears to reduce the risk of HIV injection by approximately 50% (RR 0.45, 95%CI 0.35 to 0.59, moderate-quality evidence) and there is a similar reduction in seroconversion rates (RR 0.36, 95%CI 0.19 to 0.66, low-quality evidence) compared to withdrawal or no treatment. No studies were found that compare methadone with naltrexone treatment.

Buprenorphine versus withdrawal or placebo

The Cochrane review of buprenorphine identified one study comparing buprenorphine with placebo[109], and one study comparing 1 mg per day with higher doses[110]. Compared to placebo (including 1 mg dose as placebo), buprenorphine leads to a dose-responsive reduction in heroin use and improved retention in treatment. A dose of 16 mg buprenorphine results in higher rates of retention in treatment (RR 1.52, 95%CI 1.23 to 1.88) and less morphine-positive urines (standardized mean difference (SMD) –0.65, 95%CI –0.86 to –0.44) than placebo.

Naltrexone versus placebo

The Cochrane review of naltrexone for prevention of relapse in opioid dependence identified 6 studies, with a total of 249 patients[170]. In detoxified patients, naltrexone was more effective than placebo in reducing heroin use (RR 0.72, 95%CI 0.58 to 0.90, low-quality evidence), but did not affect retention in treatment (RR 1.08, 95%CI 0.74 to 1.57) or relapse at follow-up post treatment (RR 0.94, 95%CI 0.67 to 1.34).

Safety

Methadone maintenance is associated with an increase in mortality during the first two weeks of treatment compared to pretreatment levels, due to respiratory depression[111]. After that time, there is a reduction in mortality that remains until treatment stops. Most patients will resume opioid use at some stage, and the reduction in tolerance associated with the completion of opioid withdrawal can increase the risk of opioid overdose.

Pharmacology studies suggest that buprenorphine probably has less risk of overdose than methadone, but fatal overdoses of buprenorphine combined with other sedatives can still occur.

Treatment with naltrexone may increase the risk of sedative overdose in the period following the cessation of naltrexone. Some accelerated opioid withdrawal techniques that are used to start patients on naltrexone – in particular the use of antagonists in combination with heavy sedation – also appear to increase the risk of fatal complications.

A significant proportion of patients in opioid agonist therapy develop adverse effects (see Section 6.5). Methadone leads to a slight increase in the QT interval (i.e. the time between the start of the Q wave and the end of the T wave in the heart's electrical cycle), possibly resulting in a slightly increased chance of life-threatening cardiac arrhythmias, although it is difficult to make a precise estimate of any increased risk.

Buprenorphine and naltrexone do not prolong the QT interval.

Contraindications to the use of opioid agonist maintenance treatment, and precautions for use of the treatment, include decompensated liver disease (such as with jaundice and ascites) – because in this context opioids may precipitate hepatic encephalopathy – and acute asthma and other causes of respiratory insufficiency.

Precautions for both opioid agonist treatment and opioid detoxification include high-risk polydrug use, mental illness, low levels of neuroadaptation to opioids (e.g. in recent incarceration, because many people who are incarcerated do not use opioids with the frequency required to maintain their levels of tolerance to opioids) and significant concomitant medical problems.

Precautions to the use of opioid withdrawal over agonist maintenance therapy include pregnancy (because withdrawal can lead to miscarriage), and serious acute physical or psychiatric conditions (because withdrawal may worsen or complicate management of the underlying conditions).

Cost effectiveness

In a recent study of opioid substitution therapy in different countries[112], resource-use and cost data relating to methadone and buprenorphine maintenance treatment were collected in selected WHO member states (Indonesia, Iran, Lithuania and Poland).

The total monthly cost of providing long-term methadone and buprenorphine maintenance treatment (including an initial induction phase) ranged from as little as US$26–36 in Indonesia and the Islamic Republic of Iran (approximately US$1/day) to US$296 in Poland (approximately US$10/day). This provides an indicative range within which to locate the expected investment needed to provide methadone maintenance treatment to a service user in a low or middle-income country. In high-income countries, costs for methadone and buprenorphine maintenance treatment are generally estimated to be US$5000 per year, or US$15 per day[113].

Estimation of the cost of providing medication is not an adequate basis for budgetary planning, because it may represent only a fraction of total service costs (e.g. <20% in the Islamic Republic of Iran). Studies in Australia, Canada, the United States and United Kingdom have estimated the impact of treatment on total health-care costs, social security costs, lost productivity and crime. Thus, these studies estimate the economic "return on investment" in opioid-dependence treatment[62, 114]. They show that treatment of opioid dependence pays for itself, because savings in social costs are greater than the expenditure in treatment. It is difficult to extrapolate the results of these studies to lower income countries.

Estimates of cost effectiveness in high income countries countries have found that both methadone and buprenorphine maintenance are cost effective, being well below accepted thresholds for cost–benefit analysis of treatment[115, 116].

The cost of a "one off" episode of opioid withdrawal varies significantly between settings; it depends on the method of withdrawal, the length of treatment, the medication used and staff resources.

Because of differences between maintenance and withdrawal, it is difficult to estimate the long-term cost implications of choosing between:
- opioid agonist maintenance treatment, which is low intensity and long term, and has a low relapse rate
- opioid withdrawal, which is high intensity and short term, and has a relatively high relapse rate.

Limitations of the data

No studies were found that directly compared the three different treatment approaches using a randomized design. It may be difficult to investigate this question using RCTs because patients may be reluctant to relinquish their right to choose a treatment modality. The clinical trials that were found compared the decision to attempt opioid withdrawal at one point in time versus methadone maintenance. In practice, an attempted opioid withdrawal that fails is usually followed by repeated attempts until the patient either succeeds, or stops trying to withdraw from opioids. This review found no RCTs comparing repeated attempts at opioid withdrawal with opioid agonist maintenance treatment. Also lacking were studies comparing methadone and buprenorphine maintenance treatment with opioid withdrawal and relapse prevention using naltrexone.

Treatment considerations

In practice, there is often a blurring between opioid agonist maintenance and opioid withdrawal using tapered doses of methadone or buprenorphine. Patients often start with tapering doses of agonist while trying to cease their heroin use, and increase their agonist dose temporarily whenever they relapse.

Benefits of opioid agonist maintenance treatment

The most significant benefit of opioid agonist maintenance treatment is that it has a much lower mortality rate than treatments based on opioid abstinence (the evidence for this effect is stronger for methadone than for buprenorphine). Opioid agonist maintenance treatment results in less heroin use for most patients, and better retention in drug treatment in general.

Undesirable effects and consequences

Many patients find the burden of supervised dosing every day onerous, and some patients experience adverse effects (including opioid withdrawal symptoms between doses) with methadone. Patients on methadone and buprenorphine can still experience opioid effects if they use illicit opioids; although the effects are diminished, they are not blocked completely as they would be with naltrexone. This results in good rates of retention in opioid agonist maintenance treatment, even for those people with ongoing heroin use, but it may delay the progression to long-term abstinence. Travel can be difficult for patients on methadone and buprenorphine if they are required to have their doses supervised. Unsupervised administration results in increased rates of misuse of opioid agonist medication, and diversion to illicit drug markets; also, take-home doses are occasionally consumed by children and opioid-naive adults, with fatal consequences. Cessation of methadone and buprenorphine can result in a withdrawal syndrome that is more prolonged and sometimes more severe than withdrawal from heroin. Also, many patients resume heroin use after cessation of methadone, even after long-term treatment.

Conclusion

For most patients, opioid agonist maintenance treatment will result in better outcomes than attempts at withdrawal, with or without the use of naltrexone after withdrawal. In particular, patients on opioid agonist maintenance treatment are more likely than those not undergoing such treatment to stay alive, not use heroin and be in contact with the treatment system.

> **Recommendation**
> For the pharmacological treatment of opioid dependence, clinicians should offer opioid withdrawal, opioid agonist maintenance and opioid antagonist (naltrexone) treatment, but most patients should be advised to use opioid agonist maintenance treatment.
> - Strength of recommendation – strong
> - Quality of evidence – low to moderate
> - Remarks – There is moderate evidence that agonist maintenance treatment results in less illicit opioid use in the medium term than opioid withdrawal or antagonist therapy. Opioid-dependent patients should be encouraged to use opioid agonist maintenance treatment in preference to these other approaches. There is a spectrum of severity of opioid dependence. In less severe cases of opioid dependence (e.g. non-injectors and those who have recently commenced opioid use), treatment with agonist maintenance is still recommended for most patients, but a significant number are also likely to do well with opioid withdrawal-based treatments, and it would be reasonable to recommend these to some patients.
>
> **Recommendation**
> For opioid-dependent patients not commencing opioid agonist maintenance treatment, consider antagonist pharmacotherapy using naltrexone following the completion of opioid withdrawal.
> - Strength of recommendation – standard
> - Quality of evidence – low
> - Remarks – This recommendation acknowledges that not all patients are able to access opioid agonist maintenance treatment, and that not all patients who can access it want it. In these circumstances, the use of naltrexone after withdrawal appears to have advantages over opioid withdrawal without naltrexone, in those patients who are prepared to take naltrexone.

6.3 Opioid agonist maintenance treatment

6.3.1 INDICATIONS FOR OPIOID AGONIST MAINTENANCE TREATMENT

What are the indications for opioid agonist maintenance treatment?

Agonist maintenance treatment is indicated for all patients who are opioid dependent and are able to give informed consent, and for whom there are no specific contraindications. Given the long-term nature of the treatment and the potential for toxicity in the first two weeks, a high degree of certainty of the diagnosis is required before recommending opioid agonist maintenance treatment. If the diagnosis cannot be confirmed by observation of opioid withdrawal, injection sites or confirmation of previous treatment, then treatment should be started carefully and with close monitoring; in this situation, lack of intoxication from opioid agonists will provide direct evidence of opioid tolerance. Staff should be cautious when excluding patients seeking opioid agonist maintenance treatment, because such patients often have poor clinical outcomes if they do not receive treatment[117].

6.3.2 CHOICE OF AGONIST MAINTENANCE TREATMENT

In patients to be treated with agonist maintenance treatment, should preference be given to methadone or buprenorphine?

> See evidence profile in Section A1.4 of Annex 1

Efficacy

The Cochrane Collaboration conducted a systematic review and meta-analysis on this topic in 2004[118] and updated it in 2008 (in press). Ten studies compared methadone and buprenorphine, either using flexible dosing, or doses greater than 6 mg buprenorphine or 50 mg methadone.

Flexible dose buprenorphine versus flexible dose methadone

When using flexible doses, buprenorphine was less likely than methadone to be effective in retaining patients in treatment (6 studies, 837 participants; RR = 0.82, 95%CI: 0.69 to 0.96), but there was no significant difference in heroin use based on results of morphine urinalysis (6 studies, 837 participants; SMD = –0.12, 95%CI: –0.26 to 0.02), or in terms of self-reported heroin use (2 studies, 326 participants; SMD = –0.10, 95%CI: –0.32 to 0.12).

Moderate dose buprenorphine (6–8 mg/day) versus moderate dose methadone (50–80 mg/day)

When using moderate doses, retention in treatment was better with methadone than with buprenorphine (RR = 0.79, 95%CI 0.64 to 0.99, moderate-quality evidence). Also, there was more heroin use with buprenorphine, as shown by morphine positive urines (3 studies, 314 participants: SMD = 0.27, 95%CI 0.05 to 0.50). There was no difference in self-reported heroin use (2 studies, 74 participants; SMD = –0.02, 95%CI –0.48 to 0.45).

Safety data

As a partial agonist, buprenorphine has a better pharmacological safety profile than methadone. Data on safety from randomized trials do not show significant differences between methadone and buprenorphine because of the small sample sizes. The strongest data for improved safety of buprenorphine comes from the widespread introduction of buprenorphine in France in 1995, which was followed by a 79% reduction in opioid overdose mortality[119]. From 1994 to 1998, there were an estimated 1.4 times more deaths related to buprenorphine than to methadone, although 14 times more patients received buprenorphine than methadone[120].

Although deaths have been reported where buprenorphine has been used in combination with other sedatives[121, 122], the rate of buprenorphine-related deaths is estimated at 0.2 per 1000 patient years[123], which is much less than the mortality of untreated heroin dependence[124].

In RCTs, safety data is rarely well collected; however, buprenorphine patients have been found to report more headaches, and methadone patients greater sedation[125]. There is a trend for better psychomotor performance with buprenorphine[126, 127]. When injected, buprenorphine damages veins, and complications of buprenorphine injection are common where buprenorphine is administered to injecting drug users[119, 128]. Methadone appears to prolong the QT interval, and cardiac arrhythmia adverse events have been reported. In clinical trials, the extent to which methadone prolongs the QT interval is minimal; however, there appears to be a small increase in the risk of life-threatening cardiac arrhythmias with methadone that is absent with buprenorphine [129, 130, 131, 132].

Buprenorphine tablets have a high potential for abuse. Wherever buprenorphine has been prescribed to injecting drug users, there has been an associated epidemic of buprenorphine injecting, with patients presenting for treatment using buprenorphine as their first and primary drug of abuse. While some methadone injection occurs, this is rare – particularly when take-home doses are given diluted to 200 ml per dose – and it can be managed by supervised dosing of methadone.

Supervising the dosing of buprenorphine does not completely remove the problem of abuse because it is difficult to adequately supervise the dosing of a sublingual medication that can take up to 15 minutes to dissolve. Injection of diverted buprenorphine can fuel ongoing dependence, transmit bloodborne viruses and result in fatal overdose when the drug is combined with other sedatives. It has also resulted in hepatitis, local and systemic infections, venous and arterial damage, and other injection-related problems.

Common buprenorphine-related adverse effects include headache, constipation, sleep disorders and anxiety. Buprenorphine does not appear to induce significant QT prolongation.

Overall, while buprenorphine itself is likely to be a safer medication, the difficulty of quantifying these benefits and comparing them with the risks of diversion and injection of buprenorphine mean that no conclusions on safety differences can be drawn.

Cost effectiveness

The cost of methadone is approximately US0.5–1.0 cents/mg, or US60 cents to US$1.20 per effective dose (see next section). The cost of delivery and associated treatments varies from US$5000 per annum in well-resourced countries to approximately US$500 per annum in less well-resourced countries.

Buprenorphine costs approximately US10 cents to US$1/mg, or US80 cents to US$8 per minimum recommended dose (see next section). Other costs of treatment are likely to be similar to those for methadone when buprenorphine is supervised.

Methadone is cheaper and more effective than buprenorphine at the doses studied; therefore, it is dominant in cost-effectiveness comparisons in this review.

Limitations of the data

As methadone and buprenorphine are both dose-dependent treatments, adequate comparison depends on doses. Also, because buprenorphine is a partial agonist, it is difficult to directly compare doses with methadone. Pharmacological evidence would suggest that 6–8 mg may not be the optimal buprenorphine dose. Higher doses of buprenorphine will be more effective because they act over a longer time and are more effective in blocking the effects of heroin use. Many studies have not used intention-to-treat analyses, and the patients who drop out of treatment are generally not followed up.

Treatment considerations

Methadone is available in several forms – injectable, oral solution and tablet. The oral solution form is recommended for the treatment of opioid dependence because its administration is more easily supervised; also, take-home medication is less likely to be injected when it is sufficiently diluted (e.g. to 200 mL) when administered.

Buprenorphine is a sublingual tablet most commonly available in sizes of 2 and 8 mg. Because it takes 5–15 minutes to completely dissolve, its ingestion is difficult to supervise. On the positive side, because of its long duration of action, buprenorphine can be administered every second or third day in about two thirds of patients, reducing the need for daily supervision. A formulation of buprenorphine combined with naloxone in a 4:1 ratio is also now available in Australia, Europe and the United States (see Annex 4 for further discussion).

When patients have a history of injecting buprenorphine (either illicitly obtained or prescribed), methadone maintenance should be used in preference to buprenorphine.

Other research and basic research findings

The half-life of methadone is highly variable, and a significant minority of patients will not tolerate 24-hourly methadone without withdrawal symptoms between doses[133]. For many of these patients, buprenorphine may be a better option.

Conclusion

In studies to date, methadone at standard doses has been more effective in retaining people in treatment and reducing heroin use than buprenorphine at standard doses; also, methadone is cheaper. This evidence comes from meta-analyses of well conducted clinical trials (moderate-quality evidence); however, use of higher doses of buprenorphine may produce different results. Although buprenorphine treatment might be expected to be safer than methadone treatment, this has not been confirmed by research. Currently, high-quality methadone provision should be considered the optimal treatment, with buprenorphine reserved for second-line therapy for patients in whom methadone is unwanted, inappropriate or ineffective. Patients who inject buprenorphine should be prescribed methadone in preference to buprenorphine. This conclusion places a high value on treatment outcomes over possible safety differences, because of the high mortality from untreated opioid dependence.

> **Recommendation**
> For opioid agonist maintenance treatment, most patients should be advised to use methadone in adequate doses in preference to buprenorphine.
> - Strength of recommendation – strong
> - Quality of evidence – high
> - Remarks – Although the general preference may be for methadone over buprenorphine, some patients may do better with buprenorphine. Reasons for use of buprenorphine may include previous response to buprenorphine or lack of response to methadone, short duration of action of methadone (i.e. withdrawal symptoms between doses), interaction between methadone and other medications taken, specific adverse effects of methadone, treatment availability and patient preference for subjective effects of buprenorphine compared to methadone. Reasons not to use buprenorphine include a history of buprenorphine injection, buprenorphine-specific adverse effects and failure of buprenorphine treatment in the past.

6.3.3 INITIAL DOSES OF OPIOID AGONIST MAINTENANCE TREATMENT

What initial doses of methadone or buprenorphine should be used?

Initial dose of methadone

The initial dose of methadone should be based on a careful assessment of the degree of neuroadaptation of the patient. The first two weeks of methadone treatment is a high-risk period for overdose, because it can be difficult to assess with certainty the level of neuroadaptation. For patients on prescribed opioids, the total daily dose should be converted to an equivalent methadone dose given once daily. For patients using street opioids (e.g. heroin), methadone doses of 20 mg a day will typically be adequate to relieve withdrawal symptoms and retain patients in treatment, while at the same time having a low risk of opioid overdose. Patients with low or uncertain degree of neuroadaptation should start on low doses of methadone and be closely observed. Some patients with high levels of neuroadaptation will experience some discomfort if ceasing heroin and commencing methadone at 20 mg daily. In this group, the use of higher doses (up to 30 mg) to retain patients in treatment and at greater comfort should be balanced against the risk of fatal overdose if the level of neuroadaptation is overestimated. A safer but more labour-intensive strategy is to provide an initial safe dose and review the patient several hours later to assess the response to that dose, adjust the next daily dose and, if necessary, provide a supplementary dose.

Once it has been established that the initial dose is well tolerated, the methadone dose should be gradually increased until the patient is comfortable and not using heroin or other illicit opioids. The rate of increase should be individually assessed, and should generally not be greater than 10 mg every few days.

> **Recommendation**
> During methadone induction, the initial daily dose should depend on the level of neuroadaptation; it should generally not be more than 20 mg, and certainly not more than 30mg.
> - Strength of recommendation – strong
> - Quality of evidence – very low

Initial dose of buprenorphine

The risk of overdose during buprenorphine induction is low. In patients with high neuroadaptation to opioids, however, buprenorphine may precipitate withdrawal symptoms initially, and such patients may benefit from lower initial doses (2 mg). In addition, patients should wait until they are experiencing mild opioid withdrawal before taking the first dose of buprenorphine (generally at least 12 hours since last heroin or other short-acting opioids), to reduce the risk of withdrawal symptoms precipitated by buprenorphine. Patients with moderate levels of neuroadaptation will generally tolerate initial doses of 4–8 mg a day.

Once it has been established that the initial dose is well tolerated, the buprenorphine dose can be increased fairly rapidly to a dose that provides stable effects for 24 hours and is clinically effective.

6.3.4 FIXED OR FLEXIBLE DOSING IN AGONIST MAINTENANCE TREATMENT

Should methadone and buprenorphine doses by fixed or individually tailored?

No studies were identified comparing fixed and flexible doses for methadone or buprenorphine maintenance treatment. Flexible dosing schedules are thought to be preferable because of individual differences in absorption and metabolism, and dose-related differences in clinical response. In general, the dose of methadone and buprenorphine should be increased until illicit opioid use ceases. Thereafter, the dose should be reviewed frequently, without allowing patients to become obsessed with minor changes in their dose. The methadone dose should be reviewed more frequently during induction and dose increases, after missed doses and during dose reduction. In general, the patient should be reviewed at least monthly during the maintenance phase of treatment.

6.3.5 MAINTENANCE DOSES OF METHADONE

What maintenance doses of methadone and buprenorphine should be used?

> See evidence profile in Section A1.5 of Annex 1

There is moderate-quality evidence that high doses of methadone (>60 mg) result in better retention in treatment and less heroin use than lower doses (<40 mg). Health professionals should prescribe effective doses of methadone and be prepared to increase the dose if patients are still using illicit opioids.

Fixed-dose methadone studies were divided into studies that compared 1–39, 40–59, 60–109 and above 109 mg (patients in this latter category all received 160 mg).

Efficacy

60–109 mg versus 1–39 mg

When compared to doses in the range 1–39 mg, 60–109 mg doses resulted in better retention in treatment (RR 1.36, 95%CI 1.13 to 1.63, high-quality evidence) and had higher rates of opioid abstinence (RR 1.59, 95%CI 1.16 to 2.18, low-quality evidence) and cocaine abstinence (RR 1.81, 95%CI 1.15 to 2.85, moderate-quality evidence).

60–109 mg versus 40–59 mg

When compared to doses in the range 40–59 mg, 60–109 mg doses resulted in better retention in treatment in the long term (RR 1.23, 95%CI 1.05 to 1.45, high-quality evidence), and a non-statistically significant reduction in heroin use (RR 1.51, 95%CI 0.63 to 3.61, low-quality evidence).

40–59 mg versus 1–39 mg

There was no demonstrable difference between medium (40–59 mg) and low doses (1–39 mg) in terms of retention in treatment (RR 1.26, 95%CI 0.91, 1.75, in favour of medium doses, moderate-quality evidence).

Doses above 109mg

When compared to doses in the range 60–109 mg, 160 mg per day did not result in better treatment retention (RR 0.96, 95%CI 0.69 to 1.34, low-quality evidence), although this higher dose resulted in better retention in treatment than doses below 60mg (RR 1.67, 95%CI 1.05 to 2.66).

Non-randomized studies

Numerous non-randomized studies have identified better outcomes for patients on high methadone doses[134, 135, 136, 137, 138, 139].

Safety

High methadone doses may be associated with increased risk of QT prolongation. The precise risk of QT-related adverse effects is difficult to quantity, but it is probably smaller than the benefits of high methadone doses. This is supported by the evidence for lower mortality risk for patients on high methadone doses[140].

Cost effectiveness

No studies were found that compared the cost effectiveness of high and low doses of methadone. In well-resourced countries, the cost of methadone is a small part of the overall cost of treatment, and using high doses is likely to increase the cost-effectiveness of methadone. In less well resourced countries, where the cost of methadone may make up a substantial portion of the costs of treatment, the situation is less clear. However, if heroin use is ongoing at any given methadone dose, increasing the methadone dose is likely to be a cost-effective response.

Limitations of data

The quality of the evidence on this issue is not high. Specifically, there is a lack of research of the impact of methadone doses from RCTs. Although there is a strong association between high methadone doses and good clinical outcomes based on evidence from non-randomized studies, this finding may be biased by patients who respond to methadone staying in treatment longer and on higher doses rather than is the case with those who do not respond.

Treatment considerations

In clinical practice, doses are individually tailored, based on ongoing heroin use, withdrawal symptoms between doses and adverse effects. Pharmacokinetic studies indicate large differences in methadone absorption and metabolism. In this context, trough methadone levels, measured 24 hours after dosing, are likely to be a better measure of the active dose. Some patients are likely to be adequately treated with low doses; others may need doses above the target dose range.

Conclusion

Doses in the range of 60–109 mg are more effective than lower doses. Clinicians should be encouraged to aim for doses in this range in general. Clinicians should encourage patients to use these high doses and not reduce their dose, particularly when they are still using illicit opioids.

> **Recommendation**
> On average, methadone maintenance doses should be in the range of 60–120 mg per day.
> • Strength of recommendation – strong
> • Quality of evidence – low

6.3.6 MAINTENANCE DOSES OF BUPRENORPHINE

Efficacy

No systematic reviews of the effectiveness of buprenorphine at different doses were found. In randomized trials that have been conducted comparing doses, 6 mg has resulted in less heroin use than 2 mg[141], 8 mg/day has been shown to have better retention than 3 mg per day[142] and 12 mg/day has resulted in less heroin use than 4 mg/day[143]. Two studies examining higher doses have shown a trend (not statistically significant in either study) for 16 mg to be more effective than 8 mg daily[110, 144].

Safety

Buprenorphine dose does not appear to have implications for safety. However, there is a suggestion from one RCT that alanine transaminase (ALT) and aspartate transaminase (AST) levels are more likely to be elevated in patients on higher doses of buprenorphine.

Cost effectiveness

No studies covering cost effectiveness of different doses of buprenorphine were identified in this review. The cost of buprenorphine is a significant component of buprenorphine treatment and, while higher doses are likely to be more effective, the cost effectiveness is not clear.

Limitations of the data

There are few data comparing low doses to those above 6 mg.

Other evidence

High doses of buprenorphine (16–32 mg) block the additional effects of heroin better than lower doses[145, 146, 147, 148, 149, 150] and last for longer without inducing significant additional sedation.

Conclusion

Although the quality of evidence is low, higher doses are likely to result in better retention and less heroin use than lower doses, with minimal adverse consequences other than cost. On average, doses should be at least 8 mg per day. If patients are continuing to use illicit opioids, consideration should be given to increasing the dose by 4–8 mg, to a limit of 32 mg daily.

> **Recommendation**
> Average buprenorphine maintenance doses should be at least 8 mg per day.
> • Strength of recommendation – standard
> • Quality of evidence – very low

6.3.7 SUPERVISION OF DOSING IN OPIOID AGONIST MAINTENANCE TREATMENT

Should opioid agonist maintenance treatment doses be supervised?

There has been very little systematic research on the supervision of dosing in opioid agonist maintenance treatment. All of the clinical trials demonstrating the efficacy and safety of methadone and buprenorphine against placebo or opioid withdrawal have been conducted using supervised administration, as have trials comparing methadone and buprenorphine. Non-supervised administration is used in some countries for buprenorphine treatment, most notably France, and some countries have limited supervision of dosing (such as once a week or less) for stable methadone patients. Diversion occurs with both methadone and buprenorphine if they are unsupervised, although there appears to be much greater diversion and injection of buprenorphine, even when combined with naloxone, than of methadone[151].

This is probably due to multiple factors.
- Buprenorphine is an attractive drug for injection because it produces strong effects, even in low doses, resulting in a group of individuals using buprenorphine as their first and main drug of abuse.
- The milder withdrawal symptoms with reduced buprenorphine dosing mean that patients can take some of their own buprenorphine and divert the remainder without experiencing strong withdrawal symptoms.
- Buprenorphine is difficult to supervise effectively because it is sublingually administered, taking 5-15 minutes to dissolve, wheras methadone is swallowed.

Methadone is difficult to divert when dosing is supervised and when given in diluted form (i.e. 200 mL) for take-home use its injection is rare. It has a long duration of action, making it less attractive to inject regularly. People who do purchase methadone illicitly generally use it for self treatment purposes[152].

The data on diversion and overdose deaths consistently indicate that unsupervised methadone is a hazard, because it results in a substantial number of overdose deaths in people for whom it is not prescribed[153]. Diverted buprenorphine, on the other hand, is less likely to result in death (although deaths have occurred in combination with other sedatives); however, it is likely to be injected. The main problem with buprenorphine diversion is the creation of a group of people primarily dependent on illicit buprenorphine, who are at risk from the problems associated with buprenorphine injection, which can lead to hepatitis C, HIV, endocarditis and local infections. Whether an epidemic of diverted buprenorphine is a net benefit or harm is not easy to ascertain, because it may result in a corresponding drop in heroin use; however, it would not be acceptable in many countries, because it would threaten the viability of the drug treatment system.

These points form the public health argument for supervision of treatment. On the other hand, unsupervised treatment is cheaper to set up and easy to expand. Expansion of treatment is a high priority in many areas where HIV in injecting drug users is a problem and current rates of treatment are low. Rapid expansion of unsupervised buprenorphine is argued to be the most feasible method of meeting the unmet need for treatment in the short term[154]. However, it is not clear whether unsupervised buprenorphine treatment, with its associated problems of buprenorphine injecting, would reduce HIV spread to the extent that has been demonstrated for supervised methadone treatment.

The impact of supervision of treatment on patients

themselves must be considered. Opioid dependence implies a lack of control over opioid use; thus, there are strong theoretical reasons why – at the start of treatment at least – supervision of methadone and buprenorphine may be advantageous to the patient. Unfortunately, there is a lack of clinical trial data on this topic. Research has tended to focus on patients who have been in treatment for some time, examining the impact of providing unsupervised treatment to those who meet certain criteria of stability. In this situation, RCTs demonstrate that making unsupervised treatment contingent upon cessation of illicit drug use results in a reduction in illicit opioid use.

On balance, initiating treatment with supervised dosing, assessing response to treatment, and subsequently allowing unsupervised doses to patients who demonstrate stability appears to substantially reduce diversion, probably does not diminish efficacy and is supported by patient groups.

The key elements of "stability" appear to include housing, employment, not being dependent on multiple drugs and ceasing to inject after entering treatment.

It has been argued that because the risk of overdose on buprenorphine is lower then that of methadone, and because unsupervised doses are cheaper to provide and readily accepted by patients, that in places where opioid agonist treatment is not currently available, the greatest public health benefit would occur from the introduction of buprenorphine with unsupervised dosing. It is not possible based on the current data to draw firm conclusions on this proposition. The potential benefits of making treatment more accessible, affordable and possibly more attractive to patients need to be balanced against risk of less effective treatment, creation of an illicit buprenorphine market and potential community antagonism.

Practical considerations

Supervised methadone dosing involves first dispensing methadone liquid into a clean cup, the liquid is then consumed under the direct observation of a nurse, pharmacist or doctor. Talking to patients after they have consumed their methadone is generally adequate to ensure that the dose has been taken.

Buprenorphine supervision is more difficult, because the tablet can easily be sequestered in a corner of the mouth as it takes up to 15 minutes to dissolve. The tablet should be dispensed into a clean container and tipped into the mouth of the patient, under the tongue. Periodic examination should reveal the tablet in various stages of dissolution.

If no longer needed, for whatever reason, unconsumed unsupervised doses should be returned to the place where they were dispensed.

Conclusions

On balance, initiating treatment with supervised dosing, assessing the response to treatment and subsequently allowing unsupervised doses to patients who demonstrate stability appears to substantially reduce diversion, probably does not diminish treatment efficacy and is supported by patient groups. Routine supervision of dosing with methadone or buprenorphine is recommended for all patients unless they have demonstrated that they meet commonly accepted criteria for take-home doses, developed at a regional or national level.

Recommendation
Methadone and buprenorphine doses should be directly supervised in the early phase of treatment.
- Strength of recommendation – strong
- Quality of evidence – very low

Recommendation
Take-away doses may be provided for patients when the benefits of reduced frequency of attendance are considered to outweigh the risk of diversion, subject to regular review.
- Strength of recommendation – standard
- Quality of evidence – very low

6.3.8 OPTIMAL DURATION OF OPIOID AGONIST TREATMENT

What is the optimal duration of opioid agonist treatment?

There is little research on the optimal duration of opioid agonist treatment. Studies comparing short-term opioid agonist treatment (i.e. weeks to months) to longer term treatment (6–12 months) find better results for longer term treatment. This is consistent with opioid dependence being a longer-term disease. No RCTs comparing longer treatment durations were found. Observational studies indicate that those who remain in long-term opioid agonist therapy are more likely to stay alive than those who do not, and that cessation of opioid agonist maintenance treatment is associated with a risk of relapse to opioid use. Given these findings, these guidelines recommend that opioid agonist treatment should be seen as open ended, and should be continued as long as clinically indicated. Patients and clinical staff should not take lightly the decision to terminate opioid agonist maintenance treatment (e.g. for administrative reasons). Factors predicting successful termination of opioid agonist maintenance treatment are not well described, but are likely to include employment or other meaningful activity, abstinence from opioid and other drug use while taking opioid agonists, and changes in the psychosocial environment after starting opioid agonist treatment.

Practical considerations

The decision to stop opioid substitution therapy can be a difficult one for patients, and they often seek guidance from treatment staff. On the other hand, some patients simply make up their minds that they want to cease opioid agonist treatment. In both situations, patients should be informed of the risks of cessation of the therapy and encouraged to make healthy choices. In patients doing well on opioid substitution therapy, this can also be an occasion to consider the option of more take-home doses as an alternative to cessation of opioid substitution therapy.

6.3.9 USE OF PSYCHOSOCIAL INTERVENTIONS IN MAINTENANCE TREATMENT

Should psychosocial treatments be used in addition to pharmacological maintenance treatments?

See evidence profile in Section A1.12 of Annex 1

Efficacy

A recent Cochrane Collaboration review identified eight RCTs that addressed the issue of whether psychosocial interventions should be used in addition to pharmacological maintenance treatments. Comparing methadone plus psychosocial treatment to methadone alone, the pooled analysis found no difference in treatment retention (RR 0.94, 95%CI 0.85 to 1.02, high-grade evidence); however, heroin use was significantly reduced with the addition of psychosocial treatment (RR 0.69, 95%CI 0.53 to 0.91, high-grade evidence).

Cost effectiveness

Cost effectiveness studies in the United States found that methadone with moderate intensity psychosocial services (1–2 hours per week) are more cost effective than methadone either without psychosocial services or with high intensity services (i.e. several hours a day) [155,156,157].

Limitations of data

Studies have used different techniques, including hypnotherapy, psychotherapy, acceptance and commitment therapy, interpersonal psychotherapy, supportive–expressive psychotherapy, counselling, cognitive behavioural therapy (CBT), contingency management, dialectic behaviour therapy and comprehensive validation therapy. It is difficult to compare these interventions in meta-analyses. Contingency management studies have the most consistently positive findings, regardless of whether vouchers, take-home methadone privileges or prize draw incentives are used. It is not clear whether these interventions can be generalised to settings outside the one in which they were carried out (mainly the United States).

Conclusion

Psychosocial assistance in methadone maintenance can reduce heroin use in methadone maintenance. In the United States, such services are most cost effective if they are of moderate intensity (1–2 hours a week).

> **Recommendation**
> Psychosocial support should be offered routinely in association with pharmacological treatment for opioid dependence.
> - Strength of recommendation – strong
> - Quality of evidence – high
> - Remarks – While patients should be offered psychosocial support, they should not be denied agonist maintenance treatment should they refuse such support.

6.4 Management of opioid withdrawal

Although distressing, the opioid withdrawal syndrome is rarely life threatening; however, pharmacologically assisted management of opioid withdrawal can make withdrawal from opioids more comfortable and more likely to succeed. Given the high rate of relapse, assisted opioid withdrawal is not considered an effective treatment of opioid dependence on its own (see section 6.3).

6.4.1 SIGNS, SEVERITY AND TREATMENT PRINCIPLES

The severity of opioid withdrawal depends on the dose and pharmacological properties of the opioids used, and on the extent of neuroadaptive changes that have taken place in the patient. Drugs with short half-lives will give rise to withdrawal symptoms at an earlier phase than those with long half-lives; the symptoms will also peak and resolve earlier. Untreated heroin or morphine withdrawal typically reaches its peak 36–72 hours after the last dose, and symptoms will have subsided substantially after 5 days. Untreated withdrawal from methadone or other long-acting opiates typically reaches its peak at 4–6 days, and symptoms do not substantially subside for 10–12 days. Untreated buprenorphine withdrawal following the abrupt cessation of long-term buprenorphine treatment emerges within 3–5 days of the last dose, and mild withdrawal features can continue for several weeks.

Opioid antagonists (e.g. naltrexone), which induce rapid changes in receptor activity, can precipitate withdrawal symptoms of greater severity than those normally seen in heroin withdrawal, if administered in close connection with opioid use. Treatment with naltrexone can be started within one week of cessation of short-acting opioids and buprenorphine. By contrast, naltrexone is usually not started until 10–14 days after the cessation of methadone.

The severity of withdrawal is related to the degree and rate of reversal of neuroadaptive changes related to opioid use. The most severe withdrawal occurs with the sudden reversal of significant levels of neuroadaptation; for example, when naltrexone is taken by patients who are taking high doses of methadone.

6.4.2 ASSESSMENT OF OPIOID WITHDRAWAL

When assessing the severity of current opioid withdrawal features, both subjective and objective withdrawal features are relevant. Subjective withdrawal features are a more sensitive measure of opioid withdrawal, but objective signs, when present, are more reliable. For the purpose of dose titration, it is best to place greater emphasis on observable signs rather than subjective symptoms.

Symptoms and signs of opioid withdrawal and assessment of withdrawal severity are listed below – the asterisks indicate withdrawal symptoms that can be quantified by the Subjective Opiate Withdrawal Scale (SOWS):
- sweating*
- lacrimation (excessive tear formation)*
- yawning*
- feeling hot and cold*
- anorexia and abdominal cramps*
- nausea
- vomiting and diarrhoea*
- tremor
- insomnia and restlessness*
- generalized aches and pains*
- tachycardia
- hypertension*
- piloerection (gooseflesh)
- dilated pupils
- increased bowel sounds.

Severity of withdrawal symptoms can also be quantified with the Objective Opioid Withdrawal Scale (OOWS), or with a combined single objective and subjective scale such as the Clinical Opiate Withdrawal Scale (COWS) (Annex 11).

When assessing the patient for planned opioid withdrawal, including admission to a residential detoxification facility or provision of medication to manage withdrawal symptoms, it is important to complete a thorough assessment of the patient (see section 6.1). and, as appropriate, inform the patient of the estimated risks of opioid withdrawal (including the effects of subsequent relapse), as compared to opioid agonist maintenance treatment. Since withdrawal from opioids is associated with higher mortality than opioid agonist maintenance treatment, some indication of the patient's informed consent for opioid detoxification is advised. Precautions for opioid dependence include pregnancy (specifically the first and third trimesters) and current acute comorbid conditions.

6.4.3 CHOICE OF TREATMENTS FOR ASSISTING WITHDRAWAL FROM OPIOIDS

Opioid withdrawal can be managed by controlling the rate of cessation of opioids and by providing medication that relieves symptoms, or by a combination of the two.

This analysis focuses on the three approaches to assisting withdrawal from opioids that have been most widely evaluated: tapered oral methadone, tapered sublingual buprenorphine and tapered oral adrenergic alpha-2 agonists.

There are many other alternative treatments; for example:
- shorter acting oral opioids – these are not examined here due to an absence of research on their use and difficulties in enabling supervised administration, should it be required
- recently developed transdermal formulations of opioids and adrenergic alpha-2 agonists – these may have a role to play, although research is also limited at this stage
- medications to manage specific withdrawal symptoms used in combination with opioids or alpha-2 agonists (e.g. benzodiazepines for anxiety and insomnia, anti-emetics for nausea and vomiting, and paracetamol and non-steroidal anti-inflammatory drugs [NSAIDs] for muscle aches)

Detailed guidance on the use of these medications is beyond the scope of these guidelines.

What treatments should be used to assist withdrawal from opioids?

> See evidence profile in Section A1.6 of Annex 1

Efficacy

Methadone versus alpha-2 agonists

In the pooled analysis (7 studies, 577 participants), there was no significant difference between methadone and alpha-2 agonists in treatment completion (RR 1.09, 95%CI 0.90 to 1.32, moderate-quality evidence). There was no difference in rates of relapse at follow-up (intention-to-treat analysis) (RR 1.06: 95%CI 0.55 to 2.02, low-quality evidence).

Methadone versus buprenorphine

In the pooled analysis (2 studies, 63 participants), there was no significant difference in completion of treatment between methadone and buprenorphine (RR 0.88: 95%CI 0.67 to 1.15, low-quality evidence).

Buprenorphine versus alpha-2 agonists

In the pooled analysis (8 studies, 884 participants) comparing buprenorphine to alpha-2 agonists, there were higher completion rates with buprenorphine (RR 1.67, 95%CI 1.24 to 2.25, moderate-quality evidence), lower peak objective withdrawal scores (SMD –0.61, 95%CI –0.86 to –0.36, moderate-quality evidence), and lower overall self reported levels of opioid withdrawal (SMD –0.59, 95%CI –0.79 to –0.39, high-quality evidence).

Safety

Methadone has the greatest risk of over sedation, although this is reduced with the use of lower doses (<20 mg). Buprenorphine, while safer than high doses of methadone, is nonetheless potent even at low doses, and can cause significant respiratory depression when used in combination with other sedatives, including benzodiazepines, alcohol, tricyclic antidepressants, sedating antihistamines and major tranquilizers. A number of deaths have been reported involving the combination of buprenorphine with benzodiazepines and other sedatives. As a partial agonist, buprenorphine can induce precipitated withdrawal if used while heroin is still bound to receptors. This may occur on up to 10% of occasions in which buprenorphine is used for opioid withdrawal. The main adverse effect of buprenorphine is headache. Alpha-2 agonists can cause postural hypotension, which can lead to dizziness and fainting. In overdose, alpha-2 agonists induce profound bradycardia which may require intensive care treatment but is not usually fatal. Lofexidine induces less postural hypotension than clonidine; Cochrane Collaboration reviews of clinical trials detected no difference in safety.

Cost effectiveness

There are limited data to differentiate the cost effectiveness of these medications when used for opioid withdrawal. Buprenorphine and lofexidine are more expensive than methadone. Despite this, an analysis in Australia found outpatient buprenorphine to be more cost effective than outpatient clonidine [158].

Limitations of data

It is difficult to make an assessment of the relative effectiveness of withdrawal treatment from detoxification trials because of variations in practice and because participants often leave withdrawal units on the day of the last dose, before withdrawal symptoms are completed. Data on severity of withdrawal are useful to compare treatments, but are not uniformly collected and are difficult to include in meta-analysis. Furthermore, withdrawal methods vary and few studies use the same techniques.

Treatment considerations, duration of the treatment

All treatments can be used in inpatient and outpatient withdrawal settings. Methadone and buprenorphine can be administered as once-daily supervised doses, to reduce diversion and increase safety (guanfacine can also be administered once daily, although the need for supervised dosing is less with alpha adrenergic agonists). Gradual reduction of methadone and buprenorphine can reduce the severity and increase the length of opioid withdrawal. Such gradual reductions improve treatment retention but reduce the rate of successful completion of withdrawal [159].

Conclusion

- Buprenorphine is suitable for once-daily administration; it leads to less severe withdrawal and higher rates of completion than alpha-2 agonists.
- Methadone is cheaper than buprenorphine and carries no risk of precipitated withdrawal; it is suitable for use in pregnancy.
- Alpha-2 agonists can lead to shorter duration of withdrawal symptoms and shorter time to commencement of naltrexone.

All three medications listed above can be used for opioid withdrawal. Clinical trials clearly show that buprenorphine is more effective than alpha-2 agonists, and clinical experience would suggest that methadone lies somewhere between the two, even though equivalent to both in the Cochrane Collaboration reviews. Choice should depend on the individual situation, capacity to tolerate withdrawal symptoms, timeframe and patient preferences.

> **Recommendation**
> For the management of opioid withdrawal, tapered doses of opioid agonists should generally be used, although alpha-2 adrenergic agonists may also be used.
> - Strength of recommendation – standard
> - Quality of evidence – moderate
> - Remarks – Buprenorphine and methadone are both recommended in the management of opioid withdrawal. As a partial agonist with slow receptor dissociation, buprenorphine has the best pharmacological profile for use in withdrawal, reducing the risk of rebound withdrawal when opioids are ceased. While buprenorphine is probably slightly more effective, it is more expensive.
>
> *continued on next page*

recommendation continued

> The duration of the dose taper should be at least 3 days, with a taper over 5 days for buprenorphine and 10 days for methadone resulting in acceptable withdrawal symptoms during treatment and minimal rebound withdrawal symptoms on cessation of the opioid agonist. Lofexidine should be used in preference to clonidine, particularly in outpatient settings, because it has less adverse effects.

6.4.4 ACCELERATED WITHDRAWAL MANAGEMENT TECHNIQUES

Accelerated withdrawal techniques use opioid antagonists to induce withdrawal and thus complete the process more quickly. Here, the techniques are divided depending on whether they co-administer minimal or heavy sedation. Minimal sedation refers to levels that might commonly be prescribed in the management of opioid withdrawal in outpatient or residential settings, because they have a low risk of inducing respiratory depression. Heavy sedation refers to the administration of either oral or parenteral sedatives or anaesthesia that have a significant risk of inducing respiratory depression. The use of heavy sedation requires intensive monitoring and the capacity to assist respiration, such as would be provided in an intensive care setting.

Should antagonists with minimal sedation be used for opioid withdrawal?

> See evidence profile in Section A1.8 of Annex 1

Efficacy

Four studies (394 participants) were found that examined the issue of whether antagonists with minimal sedation should be used for opioid withdrawal. In the pooled analysis, there were no significant differences in rates of completion between different opioid antagonist techniques, (RR 1.26, 95%CI 0.80 to 2.00, moderate-quality evidence). No difference in relapse rates was detected (RR 0.83, 95%CI 0.52 to 1.35, low-quality evidence[160].

Safety

Data from observational studies suggest higher rates of adverse effects with the use of opioid antagonists (RR 3.7, 95%CI 0.65 to 21.32, very low-quality evidence).

Cost effectiveness

Although the use of opioid antagonists adds to the cost of medications for opioid withdrawal, the overall cost effectiveness may be greater than conventional withdrawal treatment if the duration of withdrawal treatment is reduced[158].

Treatment considerations

Naltrexone hydrochloride is available primarily as a solid oral formulation in 25 mg and 50 mg tablets. Naloxone is available as ampoules for injection, at a concentration of 0.4 mg in 1 mL, or as a prefilled syringe.

Treatment regimens

Dosing regimens used in clinical trials range from a single dose of 50 mg naltrexone daily to a graduated increase of 12.5 mg naltrexone daily. Techniques vary from a single daily dose of naloxone to the use of naloxone infusions. Other than the observation that regimens that use higher initial doses of naltrexone are associated with higher rates of delirium, it is not clear which of these approaches is more effective. Careful and continuous monitoring is necessary during the hours immediately following administration of opioid antagonists, because of the possibility of delirium, vomiting and diarrhoea. To prevent and treat excessive diarrhoea and vomiting, expensive medications, such as ondansetron and octreatide, are often required, combined with intravenous fluid replacement. Opioid antagonist withdrawal techniques should not be undertaken in patients with a history of cardiac disease, psychosis, chronic renal impairment or decompensated liver disease, or current dependence on alcohol, benzodiazepines or stimulants.

Benefits

Use of antagonists may reduce the duration of

withdrawal; thus reducing the overall severity of withdrawal and increasing the chances of successful completion. In inpatient settings where the cost of the facility is high compared to the cost of medication, this may result in significant cost savings. This technique facilitates commencement of naltrexone treatment.

Undesirable effects and consequences

Adverse effects of opioid withdrawal treatment may include a higher peak severity of withdrawal symptoms, possibly resulting in dehydration (and resulting complications such as renal failure) and delirium. Complications from excessive sedation used in managing the increase in peak withdrawal severity could include aspiration pneumonia and respiratory depression.

Conclusion

The small number of clinical trials conducted on treatments for opioid withdrawal have used a variety of approaches, making generalization difficult. Results from these trials suggest that antagonist-induced withdrawal techniques increase the severity of opioid withdrawal initially, and may increase the adverse effects of withdrawal. Given the potential for harm, there is not enough evidence of benefit to recommend the routine use of these techniques.

> **Recommendation**
> Clinicians should not routinely use the combination of opioid antagonists and minimal sedation in the management of opioid withdrawal.
> - Strength of recommendation – standard
> - Quality of evidence – very low
> - Remarks – This recommendation places a higher value on the prevention of adverse outcomes due to delirium and dehydration than on any potential for reduced duration or overall severity of withdrawal symptoms. If opioid antagonists are to be used, careful and continuous monitoring is necessary for at least 8 hours following the administration of opioid antagonists, due to the possibility of delirium, vomiting and diarrhoea, and systems should be available for identifying and managing people who become dehydrated or delirious. Opioid antagonist withdrawal should not be undertaken in pregnant women because of the risk of inducing abortion or premature labour.

Should antagonists with heavy sedation or anaesthesia be used for opioid withdrawal?

Opioid withdrawal with opioid antagonists and heavy sedation or anaesthesia is defined as withdrawal that requires monitoring of vital functions such as respiratory rate and oxygen saturation. Such withdrawal usually takes place in intensive care settings.

> See evidence profile in Section A1.9 of Annex 1

Efficacy

A recent Cochrane Collaboration review[161] identified RCTs in which ultra-rapid opioid detoxification (UROD) was compared to:
- inpatient opioid withdrawal with clonidine (two studies[162, 163])
- inpatient withdrawal with buprenorphine (one study[163])
- opioid antagonist and minimal sedation techniques (two studies[164, 165]).

Completion of treatment and commencement of naltrexone

In the pooled analysis, there was no difference in the rates of completion of treatment of naltrexone compared to either clonidine (RR 1.15, 95%CI 0.79 to 1.68, moderate-quality evidence), or buprenorphine (RR 0.82, 95%CI 0.34 to 1.97, low-quality evidence). The use of antagonists and heavy sedation resulted in higher rates of naltrexone commencement than inpatient clonidine withdrawal (RR 3.40: 95%CI 2.32 to 4.98, moderate-quality evidence), but not inpatient buprenorphine withdrawal (RR 0.97: 95%CI 0.88 to 1.07, low-quality evidence).

Relapsed at follow-up

Heavy sedation or anaesthesia made no difference in rates of heroin use at the 6 month follow-up (RR 0.97, 95%CI 0.88 to 1.08, moderate-quality evidence).

Retention in treatment at 12 months

Heavy sedation or anaesthesia made no difference to

rates of retention in treatment at 12 months (RR 0.95, 95%CI 0.69 to 1.30, moderate-quality evidence).

Safety

Higher rates of adverse effects were seen with techniques involving heavy sedation or anaesthesia (RR 3.21, 95%CI 1.13 to 9.12, moderate-quality evidence).Potential adverse effects include severe opioid withdrawal resulting in dehydration (and resulting complications such as renal failure) and delirium. Potential complications from excessive sedation include aspiration pneumonia and respiratory depression[166]. Three life-threatening adverse events occurred out of 35 participants in the heavy sedation groups, and none out of 71 participants in the non-heavy sedation groups (RR 14, 95%CI 0.74 to 264, low-quality evidence).

Cost effectiveness

Techniques using heavy sedation and anaesthesia are expensive. In an Australian analysis, these techniques did not offer any cost-effective advantages over techniques using antagonists and minimal sedation[158].

Limitations of data

Studies do not have enough numbers to accurately determine safety data. Variations in technique may result in different patterns of safety and efficacy.

Treatment considerations

At a minimum, techniques involving heavy sedation should be conducted in a setting that is suitable for managing respiratory depression, such as an intensive care or high-dependency unit. A number of patients have died when this technique has been used outside intensive care unit settings[166, 167].

Summary

Compared with use of methadone and alpha-2 adrenergic agonist treatment for opioid detoxification, use of opioid antagonists and heavy sedation may mean that it is possible to start naltrexone earlier. However, use of opioid antagonists and heavy sedation is of little benefit over buprenorphine-assisted withdrawal or use of opioid antagonists with minimal sedation. In addition, the use of opioid antagonists and heavy sedation leads to significantly higher complication rates. Given this balance, techniques combining opioid antagonists and heavy sedation are not recommended.

> **Recommendation**
> Clinicians should not use the combination of opioid antagonists with heavy sedation in the management of opioid withdrawal.
> • Strength of recommendation – strong
> • Quality of evidence – low

6.4.5 TREATMENT SETTING FOR OPIOID WITHDRAWAL

Should withdrawal from opioids be conducted in inpatient or outpatient settings?

See evidence profile in Section A1.10 of Annex 1

Efficacy

A recent Cochrane Collaboration review[168] identified one RCT that directly addressed the issue of whether withdrawal from opioids should be conducted in inpatient or outpatient settings. The review found better rates of completion of treatment for the inpatient group (RR 1.91, 95%CI 1.03 to 3.55, very low-quality evidence). There were no differences in relapse rates between inpatient and outpatient groups (RR 1.07, 95%CI 0.97 to 1.18).

Safety

There were no data to compare the safety of inpatient and outpatient withdrawal. It might be expected that inpatient withdrawal would be safer than outpatient withdrawal, but no data are available on this topic.

Cost effectiveness

Inpatient opioid detoxification is significantly more expensive than outpatient opioid detoxification.

Australian data suggest that outpatient withdrawal with buprenorphine is significantly more cost effective[158].

Limitations of data

The RCT upon which the efficacy data is based has significant flaws; as a result, the grade of evidence is low. It seems that many patients allocated to the inpatient group either refused inpatient treatment or dropped out before opioid withdrawal was arranged.

Treatment considerations

Inpatient treatment is expensive to administer because it generally requires a secure environment, 24-hour nursing care and daily medical care. Patients in opioid withdrawal are generally restless and irritable, and it can be a challenging environment in which to work. Ensuring the health and safety of the staff in residential withdrawal units requires adequate staffing and training levels.

Benefits

Opioid withdrawal in residential facilities has higher rates of success and is probably safer.

Undesirable effects and consequences

Opioid withdrawal in residential facilities is expensive and is inconvenient for many patients.

Conclusion

Inpatient detoxification appears to have higher rates of completion of withdrawal than outpatient detoxification, but there is no demonstrable difference in relapse rates. Data to estimate the relative safety of inpatient and outpatient detoxification are lacking. It is more cost effective to provide most opioid detoxification on an outpatient basis, reserving inpatient opioid detoxification for patients who:
- have previously failed to complete outpatient detoxification
- have had complications during opioid withdrawal
- have insufficient social support or comorbid medical or psychiatric conditions.

6.4.8 PSYCHOSOCIAL ASSISTANCE IN ADDITION TO PHARMACOLOGICAL ASSISTANCE FOR OPIOID WITHDRAWAL

Is psychosocial assistance plus pharmacological assistance for opioid withdrawal more useful than pharmacological assistance alone?

> See evidence profile in Section A1.13 of Annex 1

Efficacy

The pooled results of five RCTs (184 participants) indicate that combined psychosocial and pharmacological assistance results in greater rates of completion of treatment (RR 1.68, 95%CI 1.11 to 2.55, moderate-quality evidence), lower rates of relapse at follow-up (RR 0.41, 95%CI 0.27 to 0.62, moderate-quality evidence), despite a trend towards higher rates of opioid use during detoxification (RR 1.3, 95%CI 0.99 to 1.70, moderate-quality evidence). There were no differences in rates of other substance use during detoxification[169].

Treatment considerations

The types of psychological assistance provided in the studies were contingency management, community reinforcement, psychotherapeutic counselling and family therapy. The data show no clear advantage of one technique over the others, although the evidence (from four studies) is strongest for contingency management approaches combined with methadone or buprenorphine.

Benefits

Psychosocial assistance can:
- help patients to clarify their goals around their drug use
- increase patients' motivation to stop or reduce their drug use
- increase accountability for the outcomes of the attempted opioid detoxification.

In addition, psychosocial support can help to educate patients about the sort of withdrawal symptoms they will experience, provide them with useful strategies for minimizing withdrawal and help them to interpret the current withdrawal phenomena. It can also facilitate transfer to post-withdrawal treatment options, and assist with reintegration into society.

Undesirable effects and consequences

There is a theoretical risk that psychosocial interventions to assist people undertaking opioid withdrawal may inadvertently encourage people to continue with opioid detoxification instead of moving to more effective longer term interventions, such as opioid agonist maintenance treatment.

Conclusion

For those who wish to withdraw from opioids, combined psychosocial and pharmacological assistance increases the chance of successfully completing opioid withdrawal. The evidence is strongest for contingency management approaches.

> Recommendation
> Psychosocial services should be routinely offered in combination with pharmacological treatment of opioid withdrawal.
> • Strength of recommendation – standard
> • Quality of evidence – moderate

6.5 Opioid antagonist (naltrexone) treatment

Should opioid antagonist therapy be used for opioid dependence and, if so, what are the indications for use?

Naltrexone is a highly specific opioid antagonist with a high affinity for opioid receptor sites. It effectively reverses and blocks the opioid effects of lower affinity reversible agonists, such as methadone and heroin. Naltrexone hydrochloride is available by prescription in many countries as 25 and 50 mg tablets; it is also used in the treatment of alcohol dependence.

6.5.1 INDICATIONS FOR OPIOID ANTAGONIST THERAPY

> See evidence profile in Section A1.11 of Annex 1

Efficacy

Naltrexone was compared to placebo for post-opioid withdrawal (with or without psychosocial treatment). There was no effect of naltrexone on retention in treatment (RR 1.08, 95%CI 0.74 to 1.57, moderate-quality evidence). There was a reduction in heroin use with naltrexone (RR 0.72, 95%CI 0.58 to 0.90, low-quality evidence). There was no difference in relapse at follow-up (RR 0.94, 95%CI 0.67 to 1.34, very low-quality evidence). There was also a large reduction in criminal behaviour with naltrexone (RR 0.50, 95%CI 0.27 to 0.91, very low-quality evidence).

Safety

There was no difference in reported rates of adverse effects (RR 1.21, 95%CI 0.81 to 1.81). However, some observational studies have found high rates of opioid overdose in the period after ceasing naltrexone treatment.

Limitations of data

Only a small number of studies have examined naltrexone for prevention of relapse in opioid dependence.

Benefits

Naltrexone treatment results in a reduction in heroin use and criminal behaviour. Family members of opioid addicts often like naltrexone treatment because it is clear that if the patient is taking the naltrexone they are not using heroin. Also, when family members directly observe naltrexone consumption, it gives them an opportunity to become involved in the treatment of the individual. Naltrexone blocks the effects of heroin for approximately 24 hours after each 50mg dose.

Undesirable effects and consequences

Patients often cease taking naltrexone with the intention of using heroin again, and when they do so it is difficult for them to assess the dose of heroin to use, because the effects of naltrexone are wearing off. In the space of 12 hours, the same dose of heroin can be blocked or can be fatal. This may result in higher rates of unintentional opioid overdose in people ceasing naltrexone therapy.

There is a concern that naltrexone may be used as a coercive treatment. Such coercive pharmacological treatment would be unethical. Furthermore, naltrexone used in this way would not necessarily have the same efficacy as with voluntary participants.

Treatment considerations

Naltrexone is formulated in 15 and 50 mg tablets. The cost of the medication currently varies from approximately US50 cents to US$5 per tablet. Each tablet blocks the effects of heroin for 24–48 hours. Because it completely blocks the effects of heroin, naltrexone should be prescribed to those who are aiming at complete abstinence from opioids; this limits its use to a subpopulation of more motivated patients.

Other research and basic research findings

Naltrexone may be more effective when family members are involved in the treatment or directly observe the patient taking naltrexone. Clinical experiences with naltrexone vary considerably between countries, with some countries finding levels of retention similar to opioid agonists and others finding very poor rates of retention. It is possible that cultural and social differences could result in a variable efficacy and acceptability of naltrexone treatment. Clinical experience suggests that naltrexone may be more effective in patients who are motivated to abstain from opioid use – for example, professionals at risk of losing their employment, or patients who have come before the courts and risk incarceration.

Conclusion

The limited evidence available suggests that, in dependent opioid users who have withdrawn from opioids, those who take naltrexone are less likely to use heroin or engage in criminal activity than those who do not take naltrexone. Opioid dependence has a spectrum of severity and early stages of dependence may respond better to naltrexone than more severe dependence.

Retention in treatment is generally likely to be lower than opioid agonist maintenance therapy; nevertheless, in those patients who have withdrawn from opioids and are motivated to cease opioid use completely, relapse prevention efforts with naltrexone are likely to be superior to those without naltrexone.

> **Recommendation**
> For opioid-dependent patients not commencing opioid agonist maintenance treatment, antagonist pharmacotherapy using naltrexone should be considered following the completion of opioid withdrawal.
> • Strength of recommendation – standard
> • Quality of evidence – low
> • Remarks – This recommendation is based on evidence from clinical trials that there is less heroin use with naltrexone, and on clinical experience from some countries of adequate rates of retention in treatment of patients on naltrexone. There is a concern that naltrexone may be used as a coercive treatment. Such treatment would be unethical.

6.5.2 INDICATIONS FOR NALTREXONE THERAPY

Patient selection

Given the potential for overdose after relapse, opioid antagonist therapy is likely to be most useful for those with a reasonable chance of remaining abstinent (this statement is based on expert opinion). Such groups include employed patients, those who have been using drugs for only a short time (e.g. younger patients) and those under threat of legal sanctions.

Naltrexone appears to be most useful when there is a "significant other" to administer and supervise the medication; for example, a family member, close friend or, in some cases, an employer.

Patients with severe opioid dependence should be cautious taking naltrexone; also, naltrexone is not recommended for people with cirrhosis who have a Child's severity rating of C or above.

Use in pregnancy

There is limited experience of naltrexone in pregnancy, but the likelihood of congenital abnormalities is thought to be low. If a woman taking naltrexone treatment becomes pregnant, the benefits of continuing naltrexone should be weighed against possible unforeseen risks.

The role of psychosocial therapy in naltrexone treatment

As with other pharmacological treatments, psychosocial treatment should routinely also be offered. There are insufficient data to make recommendations about specific psychosocial approaches for use in combination with naltrexone therapy; however, contingency management with vouchers has been found to be useful in maintaining abstinence and retention in treatment for patients on naltrexone[171]. In a second study, a structured group-counselling approach gave no better outcomes than optional unstructured individual counselling control group[172]. One study comparing individual counselling plus naltrexone to family counselling plus naltrexone found family counselling to be superior both during treatment and at 12 months follow-up[173].

6.6 Psychosocial interventions

The term "psychosocial support" is used here to refer to a broad range of interventions at a social and psychological level. Interventions at a social level include assistance with basic needs such as food, clothing, accommodation and employment, as well as basic health-care, friendship, community and the pursuit of happiness. Interventions at a psychological level range from unstructured supportive psychotherapy and motivational interviewing techniques, to highly structured psychological techniques. Clinicians and health providers should choose which psychosocial intervention to offer to opioid-dependent patients, based on research evidence, how appropriate a method is to the patient's individual situation, how acceptable it is to the patient, whether trained staff are available, and cultural appropriateness.

6.6.1 PSYCHOLOGICAL INTERVENTIONS

A complete discussion of the range of psychological interventions is beyond the extent of this document; however, two subtypes of therapy dominate the literature – CBT and contingency management.

CBT has become the leading approach in a variety of mental and behavioural disorders including phobias, anxiety and obsessive-compulsive disorders; it can also be effective in depression and eating disorders. CBT in substance dependence is based on the principle that addictions are learned behaviours that can be modified. Cognitive approaches primarily aim to change addictive behaviours by changing faulty cognitions that serve to maintain behaviour, or by promoting positive cognitions or motivation to change behaviour. Commonly used variants are cognitive therapy and motivational-enhancement therapy.

Behavioural approaches aim primarily to modify behaviours underpinned by conditioned learning; that is, by classical and operant conditioning. They include interventions that aim to extinguish classically conditioned responding (e.g. cue exposure and response prevention), or that are based on instrumental conditioning (e.g. community reinforcement or contingency management) – an approach in which positive non-drug taking behaviours are rewarded. Behavioural approaches involving aversive conditioning are historically important, mainly in the alcohol treatment field, but their use has ceased, mainly for ethical reasons. CBT requires training of staff in, for example, clinical psychology.

Contingency management rewards or punishes specific types of behaviours using a structured, transparent approach that increases learning of desired behaviours. Most programmes focus on positive behaviours, with reinforcement for the desired behaviour. The elements of a contingency management programme are:

- clear definitions of the desirable behaviour (e.g. opioid abstinence);
- regular monitoring for the presence or absence of the desired behaviour (e.g. regular urine tests);
- specified rewards for the desired behaviour (e.g. money, vouchers, take-home methadone doses or lottery tickets);
- positive personal feedback from staff for the desired behaviour.

Contingency management can be administered by staff with relatively little training.

Counsellors should be aware of links to available social services or other social resources in the community.

6.6.2 SOCIAL INTERVENTIONS

Vocational training

Vocational training includes a range of programmes designed to help patients find and retain employment. Vocational training can include skills training, sheltered work environments and monitoring of drug use during employment[174, 175, 176].

Housing

Housing services can vary from group accommodation for the homeless to more stable, affordable, long-term accommodation. The importance of housing is such that assistance with housing may be necessary before cessation of drug use can be attempted. While there may be risks in accommodating drug users together in institutional settings, stable accommodation in a drug-free environment is desirable. The strategies adopted will depend on local resources and norms.

Activities

The ability of patients to participate in and enjoy leisure activities of their choice is an important aspect of psychosocial support. Programmes can provide access to a range of healthy leisure activities.

Self-help groups

In the context of opioid dependence, self-help groups are voluntary, small-group structures formed by peers to assist each other in their struggle with opioid dependence. Usually abstinence oriented, they often provide both material assistance and emotional support, and promulgate an ideology or values through which members may attain a greater sense of personal identity[177].

Patients receiving pharmacological treatment should be encouraged to participate in self-help groups. Although there has been little research on this form of treatment, observational studies on 12-step groups (e.g. Narcotics Anonymous) are positive, with strong "in-treatment" effects. This form of therapy is inexpensive and provides important psychosocial support.

Social skills training

Social skills training refers to methods that use the principles of learning theory to promote the acquisition, generalization and durability of skills needed in social and interpersonal situations. Training should take place in the context of real everyday life experiences, not in closed, unrealistic settings.

Traditional healers

Traditional and spiritual healers may have a role in the provision of psychosocial support, if they are culturally acceptable to the patient. Although the assessment of these methods is beyond the scope of this document, clinical staff might wish to explore what options there are for such support with their patients.

6.6.3 PROVISION OF PSYCHOSOCIAL SUPPORT

Staff and volunteers can provide psychosocial support commensurate with their level of expertise. As a minimum, anyone providing psychosocial support to people with opioid dependence should participate in a brief training programme so that they do not put themselves at risk or inadvertently cause harm. Professional staff without specific psychotherapeutic training might be expected to be able to provide supportive psychotherapy or structured therapy based on an appropriate manual after a brief training period (e.g. 1–2 weeks).

6.7 Treatment of overdose

Opioid overdose is identifiable by a combination of signs and symptoms, including pinpoint pupils and respiratory depression. Dilated pupils suggest an alternative diagnosis. Patients with suspected opioid overdose should be treated if the respiratory rate is less than 10 per minute or if they are hypoxic on pulse-oxymetry (oxygen saturation <92%).

Initial treatment of hypoxic patients should include supplemental oxygen and assisted ventilation, as necessary. This would typically include clearing the airway and applying bag and mask ventilation with oxygen.

Naloxone is a non-selective, short-acting opioid receptor antagonist that has a long clinical history of successful use for the treatment of overdose. It is an effective antidote for overdoses of short-acting opiates such as heroin. In managing opioid overdoses, the primary concern should always be respiration and oxygenation. Any respiratory arrest should be managed with assisted ventilation and oxygen while waiting for naloxone to be administered or to take effect. Typically, adequate respiration will resume within 30 seconds of naloxone administration. The ideal dose of naloxone is one that improves ventilation without inducing withdrawal. If in doubt, it is better to err on the side of too high rather than too low a dose. A standard dose for the treatment of suspected heroin overdose is 400 mcg intramuscularly or 800 mcg subcutaneously, repeated 2 minutes later, if necessary. If there is IV access and adequate patient ventilation, small aliquots of 100 mcg can be given in repeated doses until the patient is breathing with a rate of greater than 10 breaths a minute, without inducing opioid withdrawal.

Initial use of doses of naloxone that are too high (>2 mg) can induce severe withdrawal, with the risk of vomiting and aspiration; very high doses (>10 mg) may even be life threatening[178].

Overdoses of long-acting opioids are more difficult to manage. In this situation, the duration of sedation will outlast the effects of naloxone. The safest method of treating long-acting opioid overdose is likely to be ventilation, if available. Although patients can also be managed with repeated boluses of naloxone or naloxone infusions, death can occur if there is unnoticed interruption to the naloxone infusion, or if the patient wakes up and discharges themselves from medical care.

Ideally, patients should be observed for 2 hours after naloxone administration before they are discharged. In practice, this can be difficult to achieve, but it is most important in patients where overdose is suspected to involve long-acting opioids.

In some countries, prefilled naloxone syringes are distributed to patients and family members, in combination with training in resuscitation[78, 79]. Although the use of naloxone by non-medical personnel is not without risks[80, 178], and may even be illegal in some countries, such use may prevent overdoses. Evaluation of such distribution systems has been positive[78,79], and naloxone distribution is likely to be an affordable approach to the prevention of opioid overdose, particularly where inexpensive prefilled syringes are available.

6.8 Special considerations for specific groups and settings

6.8.1 PATIENTS WITH HIV/AIDS, HEPATITIS AND TB

As described in section 5.6.8, opioid agonist treatment enhances adherence to treatment with anti-infective agents in patients with opioid dependence (see section 5.6.8 for a more detailed discussion).

When presented with an active drug user with TB and opioid dependence, the first priority of the treatment service should be to treat the active TB without spreading it further. If opioid dependence treatment can be commenced in a way that does not put other patients at risk, then this is ideal. Otherwise, it may be better to delay treatment until the patient is no longer infectious.

When presented with an active drug user with HIV and opioid dependence, it is simpler to delay antiretroviral treatment until the patient is stabilized on opioid substitution treatment than to attempt to start antiretroviral drugs before opioid substitution treatment. There is no need to delay antibiotic treatments such as co-trimoxazole or isoniazid, if it is indicated.

6.8.2 ADOLESCENTS

Adolescents 12–18 years old present to treatment services with the full range of opioid-dependence severity. Some adolescents may be brought to the clinic by their families, who are concerned about recent drug use that may not have reached the level of dependent use. On the other hand, many adolescents presenting to treatment services come from socially disadvantaged backgrounds, are living on the street and may have more severe dependence than many adult patients. In between these two groups is a third with dysfunctional families. Studies suggest that the earlier that substance use commences, the higher the risk of dependence and adverse health consequences[179].

Working with adolescents requires a sensitivity to the issues pertinent to adolescent health in general, because drug use is often a result of events occurring elsewhere in an adolescent's life. Assessment should be broad and should include medical, psychological, education, family and other aspects of the adolescent's life. Treatment should cover as many aspects of the adolescent's life as possible. Given their special treatment needs, adolescents with opioid dependence often benefit from special health services aimed directly at them.

Treatment approaches should accommodate adolescents, who often have higher levels of risk taking, novelty seeking and responses to peer pressure than older individuals (probably due to incomplete development of brain areas of inhibitory control). Thus, training in self-control, resilience and decision-making should be included in psychosocial interventions. To ensure that treatment is as effective as possible, the treatment programme needs to be individualised and comprehensive, and needs to take into consideration an adolescent's strengths, psychosocial supports, education, legal and medical status and history, and pattern of illicit drug use.

Recent research has provided important information about the clinical profile of opioid-dependent adolescents, and has underscored the high prevalence of comorbid psychiatric disorders among this population. Psychiatric disorders that often accompany opioid dependence include depression, post-traumatic stress disorder, conduct disorder and attention deficit hyperactivity disorder. Some of these disorders (e.g. depressive disorders) are more evident among opioid-dependent female adolescents than among their male counterparts. It is unclear to what extent existing psychiatric disorders lead to "self-medication" with opioids and other drugs among this adolescent population; however, addressing psychiatric comorbidity along with substance use is likely to lead to more effective, comprehensive care.

Adolescents may live with one or more parents, and are likely to still be in the legal custody of one or more parents. Parents may play a central role in the lives of adolescents entering substance abuse treatment, in comparison to adults entering treatment. Adolescents may thus be in need of family counselling, to improve relationships with parents or to help parents learn how to be as supportive as possible of their adolescent while that person is in treatment for their substance use disorder. High levels of parental involvement and low levels of parental detachment protect against opioid use among adolescents.

Experimentation with substance use often starts in adolescence; thus, addiction or substance dependence, has frequently been referred to as a developmental disorder. Providing effective interventions early in an adolescent's drug involvement is critical if this progression is to be altered. Early intervention is particularly important in light of emerging research, suggesting that adolescents may progress from substance use to dependence more rapidly than adults. Additionally, substance use among adolescents may interfere with cognitive, social and emotional development[15, 180].

Effective early intervention for opioid-dependent adolescents – combining pharmacotherapy and psychosocial treatment – can help to prevent adolescents from following a substance-using life trajectory, and from transitioning from intranasal or oral to injecting opioid use. Moreover, early psychosocial intervention with young people who have used heroin but who are not yet opioid dependent can help to prevent young people from becoming dependent on opioids.

Should pharmacological treatment for adolescents with opioid dependence differ from that for adults?

No systematic reviews addressing this question were found. Some clinical trials were found that supported the use of agonist pharmacotherapy, both for opioid withdrawal and maintenance. One RCT demonstrated that, compared to clonidine patches, 28-day reducing buprenorphine retained more people in treatment (72% versus 39%), and led to higher rates of induction to naltrexone (61% versus 5%)[181].

The use of agonist pharmacotherapy is still the recommended therapy for adolescent opioid dependence. However, adolescents with a short period of dependence and those living in families may respond to opioid withdrawal with or without naltrexone, and these would be reasonable alternatives. Opioid agonist pharmacotherapy in this population can also be started on an interim or trial basis, and short-term therapy may be all that is required if the response is positive.

A comprehensive treatment programme that addresses this entire clinical profile is more likely to produce better outcomes than a programme that focuses on one clinical problem in isolation.

6.8.3 WOMEN

Women have been found to differ from men in their drug-use patterns, with women using less quantity but advancing more quickly to dependence, and using more prescription sedatives. Women who become opioid dependent are more likely to have less education, fewer financial resources and higher rates of sexual and physical abuse[183]. Often, the needs of women in substance dependence treatment settings are also different. They are more likely to have child-care responsibilities that may limit access to treatment, and they may be reluctant to participate in group psychosocial activities with men. They also report significant rates of sexual harassment by male treatment staff[183].

Data are lacking on the relative efficacy of gender-specific services for women. To retain women, services may need to provide either individual or female-only group counselling, cater for people with small children (e.g. provide child-care facilities), and have measures to guard against sexual harassment of female patients by male staff.

6.8.4 PREGNANCY AND BREASTFEEDING

For women who are pregnant or breastfeeding, opioid agonist maintenance with methadone is seen as the most appropriate treatment, taking into consideration effects on the fetus, neonatal abstinence syndrome, and impacts on antenatal care and parenting of young children. Opioid-dependent women not in treatment should be encouraged to start opioid agonist maintenance treatment with methadone or buprenorphine. Pregnant women who are taking opioid agonist maintenance treatment should be encouraged not to cease it while they are pregnant. Although many women want to cease using opioids when they find out they are pregnant, opioid withdrawal is a high-risk option because a relapse to heroin use will affect the capacity to care for the child. In addition, severe opioid withdrawal symptoms may induce a spontaneous abortion in the first trimester of pregnancy, or premature labour in the third trimester. Relapse to heroin use during pregnancy can also result in poorer obstetric outcomes. Opioid agonist maintenance is thought to have minimal long-term developmental impacts on children when compared to the risk of maternal heroin use and resulting harms.

Methadone is preferred over buprenorphine because of the longer experience of the safety of methadone in pregnancy compared to buprenorphine, despite the fact that early research with buprenorphine suggests that its use may result in less neonatal abstinence syndrome than occurs with the use of methadone. If women are being successfully treated with buprenorphine, then the benefit of staying with a treatment that is working should also be taken into consideration.

In the second and third trimester, methadone doses may need to be increased, due to increased metabolism and circulating blood volume. Splitting the dose into two 12-hour doses may produce more adequate opioid replacement in this period. After birth, the dose of methadone may also need to be adjusted as some of these changes reverse.

Although methadone and buprenorphine are detectable in breast milk, the levels are low and are not thought to significantly affect the infant. Breastfeeding, on the other hand, has many benefits, including mother–infant bonding, nutrition and prevention of childhood illness. Opioid-dependent mothers should be encouraged to breastfeed, with the possible exception of HIV-positive mothers or those using alcohol or cocaine and amphetamine type drugs; in such cases, specific advice should be sought.

Untreated neonatal abstinence syndrome can cause considerable distress to infants and, in rare cases, can cause seizures. Cochrane Collaboration reviews indicate that opioids and barbiturates are more effective than placebo or benzodiazepines, with opioids probably more effective than barbiturates.

> **Recommendation**
> Opioid agonist maintenance treatment should be used for the treatment of opioid dependence in pregnancy.
> • Strength of recommendation – strong
> • Quality of evidence – very low
>
> **Recommendation**
> Methadone maintenance should be used in pregnancy in preference to buprenorphine maintenance for the treatment of opioid dependence; although there is less evidence about the safety of buprenorphine, it might also be offered.
> • Strength of recommendation – standard
> • Quality of evidence – very low

6.8.5 OPIUM USERS

People dependent on opium who are suffering harm as a result can be treated with opioid agonist maintenance treatment, consistent with the approach for dependence on other opioids. Two trials have demonstrated the effectiveness of buprenorphine in this population[184, 185].

It is important to ensure that opium smokers meet criteria for opium dependence beyond simple tolerance and withdrawal. If unclear, it may be wise for opium smokers to attempt withdrawal first before commencing opioid agonist maintenance treatment.

6.8.6 DRIVING AND OPERATING MACHINERY

Opioid intoxication can occur during induction onto methadone or buprenorphine. Patients should be advised not to drive while sedated. As patients will not know what effect their first few methadone and buprenorphine doses will have on them, they should be advised not to plan to drive at this time.

6.8.7 PSYCHIATRIC COMORBIDITY WITH OPIOID DEPENDENCE

Psychiatric comorbidity with opioid dependence is common; in particular, depression, anxiety, personality and post-traumatic stress disorders should be specifically looked for early in treatment and on a regular basis thereafter. As with medical comorbidity, there is likely to be a greater uptake of treatment if the treatment can be provided by the same medical practitioner or at the same facility in an integrated service. Failing that, strong links with other services should be established to facilitate referral and to establish the framework for joint involvement; such a framework should include clarification about prescribing of psychoactive medication and about giving the patient a consistent therapeutic message.

6.8.8 POLYSUBSTANCE DEPENDENCE

Annex 12 lists the acute and chronic interactions of opioids, alcohol, benzodiazepines, stimulants and cannabis.

In the treatment of polysubstance dependence, opioid agonist maintenance treatment can be started for the opioid dependence component, in an inpatient facility if necessary, while the person is simultaneously withdrawn from alcohol, benzodiazepines and stimulants.

For withdrawal from high doses of benzodiazepines, gradual withdrawal may be necessary. If benzodiazepines are to be given to outpatients on opioid agonist maintenance treatment, this should be done carefully, because there is little evidence to support the long-term use of these drugs and they increase the risk of sedative overdose. If gradually reducing doses of benzodiazepines are prescribed to facilitate the safe withdrawal from benzodiazepines, the prescription should be from a single practitioner, and the dispensing should occur with administration of the dose of methadone, if possible. Patients should be discouraged from withdrawing from opioid agonist maintenance before ceasing benzodiazepines.

6.9 Management of pain in patients with opioid dependence

6.9.1 ACUTE PAIN

Pain in patients with opioid dependence is often exacerbated by the lowering of the pain threshold that tolerance to opioids can induce. Opioid-dependent patients are more resistant to pain management with opioids, due either to their tolerance to opioids or to blocking effects of medications used to treat opioid dependence, including buprenorphine and naltrexone. Patients with opioid dependence have a right to adequate pain relief; however, some patients will try to manipulate the health system to obtain opioids. Measures that can be taken to minimize this include:
- managing pain through a single health service (hospital or primary care practice – depending on the severity)
- adequately defining the nature of the painful condition
- resolving acute pain rapidly, and then moving quickly to longer acting opioids that have less potential for abuse and produce stable opioid effects (as opposed to cyclical patterns of intoxication and withdrawal).

Clinical assessment should be used to distinguish between opioid withdrawal and opioid intoxication. Opioids should be titrated to pain response, with close assessment of the clinical features of withdrawal and intoxication, to determine appropriate dose levels.

Patients not on agonist maintenance treatment

For patients using illicit opioids without opioid agonist maintenance treatment, starting opioid agonist maintenance treatment with methadone allows for combined management of opioid dependence and pain. Inadequate analgesia often contributes to patients self-administering illicit opioids.

Patients on antagonist medication (naltrexone)

Patients on naltrexone will not respond to opioid analgesics in a regular manner. For mild *Pain*. non-opioid analgesics (e.g. paracetamol and NSAIDs) should be used. Patients taking naltrexone will not benefit from opioid-containing medicines such as cough, cold and antidiarrhoeal preparations. In an emergency, pain management may consist of regional analgesia; conscious sedation with non-opioids such as benzodiazepines or ketamine; and use of non-opioid techniques of general anaesthesia. For elective surgery pain management in hospital, naltrexone should be discontinued at least 72 hours before elective surgery (including dental surgery), if it is anticipated that opioid analgesia may be required. The treating surgeon or doctor should be informed that the patient has been taking naltrexone. The patient should then be abstinent from opioids for three to seven days – depending on the duration of the opioid use and the half-life of the opioid – before resuming naltrexone treatment. If in doubt, a naloxone challenge test can be administered to determine whether naltrexone can be recommenced without inducing opioid withdrawal.

Patients on partial agonists (buprenorphine)

Because of the high affinity of buprenorphine for the opioid receptor, patients treated with buprenorphine may need higher effective opioid activity to manage acute pain. The high affinity opioid agonist fentanyl may be more effective than other opioids in this situation. For mild *Pain*. increasing the dose of buprenorphine or addition of weak opioids (e.g. tramadol) may be effective, although such approaches have not been systematically investigated.

For treatment of acute pain not responding to these measures, the options are to:
- cease buprenorphine and use full opioid agonists, such as methadone or morphine, then switch back to buprenorphine when pain resolves
- continue buprenorphine with the use of high doses of opioids but, as the blocking effect of buprenorphine reduces over time, take care to avoid overdose if buprenorphine is ceased while high doses of opioids are continued
- continue buprenorphine and use non-opioid analgesia such a ketamine infusion; or employ the judicious adjunctive use of clonidine or benzodiazepines.

Patients on full agonist (methadone)

For mild or acute *Pain*, consider non-opioid analgesics (e.g. paracetamol). Where parenteral analgesics are required, the NSAID ketorolac should be considered. For elective surgery, pain management in hospital is recommended. Patients on methadone who are experiencing acute pain in hospital often receive inadequate doses of opioids for their pain. For patients in methadone maintenance treatment, the same analgesic techniques should be used in the same way as for other patients; such techniques include the use of injectable and patient-controlled analgesia. Because of their tolerance of opioids, patients taking methadone will require larger doses of opioid analgesia for adequate pain relief.

Partial agonists, such as buprenorphine, should be avoided because they may precipitate withdrawal symptoms. There is evidence of cross-tolerance between methadone and anaesthetic agents; thus, patients on methadone may require higher doses of anaesthetic agents in the event of dental or surgical procedures. Patients needing methadone for ongoing management of chronic pain benefit from a comprehensive management plan. Specialist advice should be sought regarding such patients.

6.9.2 CHRONIC PAIN

The recent escalation in the use of opioids for chronic pain in some parts of the world[186] suggests a significant overlap between treatment of chronic pain and dependence on prescription opioids. This document does not attempt to address the use of opioids in the management of chronic pain; however, patients with chronic pain and patterns of use of their prescribed opioids that fit the criteria for dependence (i.e. more than just tolerance and withdrawal), are often referred (or refer themselves) to opioid-dependence treatment facilities. Typically, they present with problems such as injecting their prescribed opioids, taking rapidly escalating doses of opioids and taking opioids in greater quantities than prescribed (resulting in intoxication or overdose); they may also present with other features that raise suspicions of misuse, which they may deny.

In the management of such patients, the first step could be to determine that there has been a comprehensive assessment of the cause of the *Pain*, both physical and psychological, with any physical cause found being treated. For patients not on opioid agonist maintenance treatment, the next step would be to provide supervised methadone or buprenorphine in place of unsupervised opioids, to provide stable opioid effects and eliminate cycles of withdrawal and intoxication. For pain persisting despite adequate opioid agonist maintenance treatment, opioid rotation should be considered.

In some cases, it could be that the opioid treatment is no longer useful, either because it is being abused or because it is suspected that pain is being exacerbated by opioid-induced hyperalgaesia[187]. Opioid withdrawal may be considered as an approach to reverse opioid-induced hyperalgaesia, although it may risk relapse to illicitly obtained opioids.

Measures that can be taken to prevent the abuse of prescription opioids include systems that encourage all opioid analgesia to be provided by one doctor, a graded approach to supervision of dosing, prescription of formulations less liable to abuse (e.g. liquid methadone formulations) and careful patient selection.

Annex 1 Evidence profiles

The following evidence profiles have been produced by applying the GRADE working group approach to determining the quality of evidence to the questions addressed. More information on this approach is contained in Section 2.

A1.1 Is methadone effective for the treatment of opioid dependence?

GRADE evidence profile

Author(s):	Amato L
Date:	23 August 2006
Question:	Should methadone maintenance treatment versus opioid withdrawal or no treatment be used for opioid dependence?
Patient or population:	opioid addicts
Settings:	outpatient
Systematic review:	Mattick RP et al. (in press) *Methadone maintenance therapy versus no opioid replacement therapy for opioid dependence* (CLIB 3, 2003)[105]; Bargagli AM et al. (2007) *A systematic review of observational studies on treatment of opioid dependence*.[197]

(Throughout this annex, −1 is used to indicate that the score has been reduced by one because of a weakness in this area).

Quality assessment						Summary of findings					
						No of patients		Effect		Quality	Importance
No. studies	Design	Limitations	Consistency	Directness	Other considerations	Methadone maintenance treatment	No treatment	Relative risk (RR) (95% CI)	Absolute risk (AR) (95% CI)		
Use of opioids (subjective follow-up: 1 month–2 years)											
3[a] [66,188,189]	Randomized trials[b]	Some limitations[b] (−1)	No important inconsistency	No uncertainty	None	28/104 (26.9%)	110/126 (87.3%)	RR 0.323 (0.23 to 0.44)	AR 630/1000 less (830 less to 430 less)	⊕⊕⊕⊖ Moderate	7
Criminal behaviour (objective follow-up: 1 month–2 years)											
3[a] [66,188,189]	Randomized trials[b]	Some limitations[b] (−1)	No important inconsistency	No uncertainty	Imprecise or sparse data (−1)	5/178 (2.8%)	18/185 (9.7%)	RR 0.393 (0.12 to 1.25)	AR 250/1000 less (700 less to 19 more)	⊕⊕⊖⊖ Low	6
Mortality from randomized controlled trials (RCTs) (objective follow-up: 2–3 years)											
3[d] [188,106,189]	Randomized trials[e]	No limitations	No important inconsistency	No uncertainty	Imprecise or sparse data (−2)	3/216 (1.4%)	7/219 (3.2%)	RR 0.493 (0.06 to 4.23)	AR 16/1000 less (100 less to 30 more)	⊕⊕⊖⊖ Low	9
Mortality (any cause) from observational studies (objective follow-up: 2.5 years–21 years)											
5[f] [190-194]	Observational studies[g]	No limitations	No important inconsistency	No uncertainty	None	257/19421 (1.3%)	1063/23614 (4.5%)	RR 0.37 (0.29 to 0.48)	AR 20/1000 less (30 less to 10 less)	⊕⊕⊖⊖ Low	9
Mortality (overdose) from observational studies (objective follow-up: 2.5 years–12 years)											
5[h] [190,191,193,195,196]	Observational studies[i]	No limitations	Inconsistent results between studies (−1)10	No uncertainty	Extremely strong effect (+2)	70/37516 (0.2%)	416/32454 (1.3%)	RR 0.17 (0.05 to 0.63)	AR 10/1000 less (20 less to 0.00)	⊕⊕⊕⊖ Moderate	9
Retention in treatment (objective follow-up: 1 month–2 years)											
3[k] [106,108,107]	Randomized trials[l]	No limitations	No important inconsistency	No uncertainty	None	173/254 (68.1%)	63/251 (25.1%)	RR 3.053 (1.75 to 5.35)	AR 460/1000 more (270 more to 650 more)	⊕⊕⊕⊕ High	7

[a] Three studies in an outpatient setting; two were conducted in the United States and one in Sweden.
[b] Three randomized controlled trails (RCTs): one with adequate allocation concealment, one unclear and one inadequate.
[c] Random effect model.
[d] Three RCTs, one conducted in the United States, one in Sweden and one in China.
[e] One adequate and two unclear allocation concealment.
[f] Five studies in an outpatient setting; conducted in Italy, Australia, Sweden, the United States and Spain (one in each).
[g] Quality of studies using Newcastle–Ottawa Scale: selection, two studies rated 3 and three studies rated 2; comparability, one study rated 3, three studies rated 1 and one study rated 0; outcome, two studies rated 2 and three studies rated 1.
[h] Five studies in an outpatient setting: two conducted in the Netherlands and one each in Italy, the United States and Spain.
[i] Quality of studies using Newcastle–Ottawa Scale: selection, four studies rated 3 and one study rated 2; comparability, two studies rated 2 and three studies rated 1; outcome, one study rated 2 and four studies rated 1.
[j] High statistical heterogeneity *P* < 0.00001, but all consistent results.
[k] Three studies in an outpatient setting, conducted in Hong Kong, Thailand and the United States (one each).
[l] Three RCTs, all with unclear allocation concealment.

A1.2 Does opioid agonist maintenance treatment reduce the spread of HIV?

GRADE evidence profile

Author(s):	Amato L, Minozzi S
Date:	22 May 2006
Question:	Should agonist maintenance treatment be used for the prevention of HIV infection or reduction of high-risk behaviours?
Patient or population:	injecting opioid dependent
Settings:	Outpatient
Systematic review:	Gowing L et al. (2004) *Substitution treatment of injecting opioid users for prevention of HIV infection* (CLIB 4, 2004)[203].

Quality assessment						Summary of findings					
						No of patients		Effect		Quality	Importance
No. studies	Design	Limitations	Consistency	Directness	Other considerations	Agonist maintenance treatment	No treatment	Relative risk (RR) (95% CI)	Absolute risk (AR) (95% CI)		
Injecting behaviour: prevalence of injecting, cohort study (subjective follow-up: 18 months)											
1[a][198]	Observational studies[b]	No limitations	No important inconsistency	No uncertainty	None	125/152 (82.2%)	97/103 (94.2%)	RR 0.87[3] (0.80 to 0.95)	AR 120/1000 less (200 less to 40 less)	⊕⊕○○ Low	6
Injecting behaviour: prevalence of injecting (subjective follow-up: 4 months)											
1[d][199]	Randomized trials[e]	No limitations	No important inconsistency	Some uncertainty (−1)[f]	None	44/129 (34.1%)	93/124 (75.0%)	RR 0.45[3] (0.35 to 0.59)	AR 410/1000 less (520 less to 300 less)	⊕⊕⊕○ Moderate	6
Injecting behaviour: proportion of patients sharing injecting equipment, observational studies (subjective follow-up: 0–18 months)											
3[g][198, 200, 201]	Observational studies[h]	No limitations	No important inconsistency	No uncertainty	None	83/301 (27.6%)	424/1020 (41.6%)	RR 0.54[c] (0.37 to 0.79)	AR 230/1000 less (400 less to 60 less)	⊕⊕○○ Low	7
Sexual behaviour: commercial sex (follow-up: 18 months)											
1[a][198]	Observational studies[i]	No limitations	No important inconsistency	No uncertainty	None	43/152 (28.3%)	47/103 (45.6%)	RR 0.62[c] (0.45 to 0.86)	AR 170/1000 less (290 less to 50 less)	⊕⊕○○ Low	7
Sexual behaviour: unprotected sex (follow-up: 3–6 months)											
2[j][198, 200]	Observational studies[k]	No limitations	No important inconsistency	No uncertainty	None	174/213 (81.7%)	554/654 (84.7%)	RR 0.94[d] (0.87 to 1.02)	AR 60/1000 less (130 less to 10 more)	⊕⊕○○ Low	6
Seroconversion to HIV (variable follow-up: up to 5 years)											
2[l][198, 200]	Observational studies	No limitations	No important inconsistency	No uncertainty	None	16/579 (2.8%)	24/297 (8.1%)	RR 0.36[c] (0.19 to 0.66)	AR 50/1000 less	⊕⊕○○ Low	8

[a] One study in an outpatient setting, conducted in the United States (Metzger, 1993)[198].
[b] One descriptive study in which the author rated the quality of the study on the basis of six items (description of the population, description of eligibility criteria, adjustment for confounding, less than 20% loss to follow-up, presence of co-intervention, inconsistency in data collection between groups) rated from 0 to 1 where 0 = no bias. On the basis of this rating system the study was rated 1.
[c] Random effect model.
[d] One study conducted in Australia, in an inpatient setting (in prison).
[e] The study was rated 1 (see footnote 2).
[f] Opioid-dependent prisoners.
[g] All three studies were conducted in an outpatient setting, two in the United States and one in Germany.
[h] Three cohort studies, two rated 1 and one 2 (see footnote 2).
[i] One cohort study rated 1 (see footnote 2).
[j] Both outpatient, one conducted in the United States and one in Germany.
[k] Both rated 1 (see footnote 2).
[l] Two cohort studies: Metzger (1993)[198] a non-treatment control group selected by methadone group, and Moss (1994)[202] a control group selected from contemporaneous entry to opioid withdrawal programme.

A1.3   Is buprenorphine effective for the treatment of opioid dependence?

GRADE evidence profile

Author(s):	Amato L, Minozzi S
Date:	23 May 2006
Question:	Should buprenorphine maintenance versus placebo be used for opioid addiction?
Patient or population:	Opioid dependent
Settings:	Outpatient and inpatient
Systematic review:	Mattick RP et al. *Buprenorphine maintenance versus placebo or methadone maintenance for opioid dependence* (2008, in press)[118].

Quality assessment						Summary of findings					
						No of patients		Effect		Quality	Importance
No. studies	Design	Limitations	Consistency	Directness	Other considerations	Buprenorphine	Placebo[e]	Relative risk (RR) (95% CI)	Absolute risk (AR) (95% CI)		
Retention in treatment: 2–4 mg buprenorphine versus placebo or 1 mg buprenorphine (objective follow-up: 2–16 weeks[d])											
2 [109, 110]	Randomized trials[b]	No limitations	No important inconsistency	One inpatient study (–1)	None	141/242 (58%)	114/245 (47%)	RR 1.24[c] (1.06 to 1.45)	AR 100/1000 more (30 more to 210 more)	⊕⊕⊕◯ Moderate	7
Morphine positive urines: 2–4 mg buprenorphine versus placebo or 1 mg buprenorphine											
2 [109, 110]	Randomized trials[b]	No limitations	Inconsistent results between studies (–1)	One inpatient study (–1)	None	242	245	–	SMD 0.10[c] (–0.8 to 1.01)	⊕⊕◯◯ Low	7
Retention in treatment: 8 mg buprenorphine versus placebo or 1 mg buprenorphine (objective follow-up: 2–16 weeks[d])											
2 [109, 110]	Randomized trials[b]	No limitations	No important inconsistency	One inpatient study (–1)	None	119/218 (54%)	114/245 (47%)	RR 1.21[c] (1.02 to 1.44)	80/1000 more (9 more to 191 more)	⊕⊕⊕◯ Moderate	7
Morphine positive urines: 8 mg buprenorphine versus placebo or 1 mg buprenorphine											
2 [109, 110]	Randomized trials[b]	No limitations	Inconsistent results between studies (–1)	One inpatient study (–1)	None	218	245	–	SMD –0.28[c] (–0.47 to -0.10)	⊕⊕◯◯ Low	7
Retention in treatment: 16 mg buprenorphine versus 1 mg buprenorphine (objective follow-up: 2–16 weeks[d])											
1 [110]	Randomized trials[b]	No limitations	No important inconsistency	No uncertainty	None	110/181 (61%)	74/185 (40%)	RR 1.52[c] (1.23 to 1.88)	210/1000 more (90 more to 350 more)	⊕⊕⊕⊕ High	7
Morphine positive urines: 16 mg buprenorphine versus placebo or 1 mg buprenorphine											
1 [110]	Randomized trials[b]	No limitations	No important inconsistency	No uncertainty	None	181	185	–	SMD –0.65[c] (–0.44 to –0.86)	⊕⊕⊕⊕ High	7

[a]   Two RCTs: one inpatient, one outpatient, both conducted in the United States.
[b]   Both with unclear allocation concealment.
[c]   Random effect model.
[d]   Length of treatment.
[e]   Placebo or 1 mg buprenorphine daily.

A1.4 Methadone versus buprenorphine

GRADE evidence profile

Author(s):	Amato L, Minozzi S
Date:	22 March 2006
Question:	Should buprenorphine maintenance flexible doses versus methadone maintenance flexible doses be used for opioid maintenance treatment?
Patient or population:	Opiate dependents
Settings:	Outpatient
Systematic review:	Mattick RP et al. *Buprenorphine maintenance versus placebo or methadone maintenance for opioid dependence* (2008, in press).[105]

Quality assessment						Summary of findings					
						No of patients		Effect		Quality	Importance
No. studies	Design	Limitations	Consistency	Directness	Other considerations	Buprenorphine maintenance flexible doses	Methadone maintenance flexible doses	Relative risk (RR) (95% CI)	Absolute risk (AR) (95% CI)		
Retention in treatment flexible doses buprenorphine versus flexible doses methadone (objective follow-up: 6–48 weeks[d])											
7[a] [68, 125, 205-209]	Randomized trials	No limitations[b]	No important inconsistency	No uncertainty	None	255/484 (52.7%)	310/492 (63.0%)	RR 0.82[c] (0.72 to 0.94)	130/1 000 (220 less to 40 less)	⊕⊕⊕⊕ High	7
Use of opioid during the treatment[g] (better indicated by: lower scores)											
6[e] [125, 205, 207-210]	Randomized trials	No limitations[f]	No important inconsistency	No uncertainty	None	411	426	---	SMD –0.12 (–0.26 to +0.02)	⊕⊕⊕⊕ High	7
Use of cocaine during the treatment[g] (better indicated by: lower scores)											
5[h] [205, 207-210]	Randomized trials	No limitations[i]	No important inconsistency	No uncertainty	None	384	395	---	SMD 0.11 (–0.03 to +0.25)	⊕⊕⊕⊕ High	5
Use of benzodiazepine during the treatment[g] (better indicated by: lower scores)											
4[j] [207-210]	Randomized trials	No limitations[k]	No important inconsistency	No uncertainty	None	329	340	---	SMD 0.11 (–0.04 to +0.26)	⊕⊕⊕⊕ High	4
Criminal behaviour (better indicated by: lower scores)											
1[l] [207]	Randomized trials	No limitations[m]	No important inconsistency	No uncertainty	Imprecise or sparse data (–1)[n]	95	117	---	SMD –0.14 (–0.41 to +0.14)	⊕⊕⊕○ Moderate	6

[a] All outpatient, country of origin: three United States, one Austria, one Switzerland, one Australia, one United Kingdom.
[b] Two studies with adequate allocation concealment, for the others five not described; 5/7 double blind.
[c] Random effect model.
[d] Length of treatment.
[e] All outpatient, country of origin: three United States, one Austria, one Australia, one Switzerland.
[f] 5/6 double blind; one adequate allocation concealment, five not stated.
[g] Data based on urinalysis.
[h] All outpatient, country of origin: three United States, one Austria, one Australia.
[i] 4/5 double blind; one adequate allocation concealment, five not stated.
[j] All outpatient, country of origin: two United States, one Austria, one Australia.
[k] 3/4 double blind; one adequate allocation concealment, five not stated.
[l] Outpatient, conducted in Australia.
[m] Double blind, adequate allocation concealment.
[n] Only one study with the results not statistically significant.

GRADE evidence profile

Author(s):	Amato L, Minozzi S
Date:	23 March 2006
Question:	Should buprenorphine maintenance moderate doses (6–12 mg/day) versus methadone maintenance moderate doses (50–80 mg/day) be used for opioid dependence?
Patient or population:	Opiate dependents
Settings:	Outpatient
Systematic review:	Mattick RP et al. *Buprenorphine maintenance versus placebo or methadone maintenance for opioid dependence* (2008, in press)[105].

Quality assessment						Summary of findings					
						No of patients		Effect		Quality	Importance
No. studies	Design	Limitations	Consistency	Directness	Other considerations	Buprenorphine maintenance high doses (6–12 mg/day)	Methadone maintenance high doses (50–80 mg/day)	Relative risk (RR) (95% CI)	Absolute risk (AR) (95% CI)		
Retention in treatment (follow-up: 17–52 weeks[e])											
7[a] [141, 143, 328-332]	Randomized trials	No limitations[b]	Important inconsistency (−1)[c]	No uncertainty	None	158/356 (44.4%)	199/352 (56.5%)	RR 0.79[d] (0.64 to 0.99)	120/1000 (230 less to 10 less)	⊕⊕⊕O Moderate	7
Use of opioids[g] (better indicated by: lower scores)											
3[f] [143, 329, 330]	Randomized trials	No limitations[h]	No important inconsistency	No uncertainty	Imprecise or sparse data (−1)	157	157	—	SMD 0.27 (0.05 to 0.50)	⊕⊕⊕O Moderate	7
Use of cocaine[g] (better indicated by: lower scores)											
1[i] [143]	Randomized trials	No limitations[a]	No important inconsistency	No uncertainty	Very imprecise or sparse data (−2)[j]	29	28	—	SMD 0.22 (−0.30 to 0.74)	⊕⊕OO Low	5

a All outpatient, six conducted in the United States, one in Italy.
b All double blind, one adequate allocation concealment, the others not described.
c High heterogeneity $P = 0.04$
d Random effect model.
e Length of treatment.
f All outpatient and all conducted in the United States.
g Based on urinalysis.
h Three double blind, one with adequate allocation concealment, the others not stated.
i Outpatient, conducted in the United States.
j Double blind, allocation concealment not stated.
k Only one study, few patients, result not statistically significant.

A1.5 What maintenance doses of methadone should be used?

GRADE evidence profile

Author(s):	Amato L, Minozzi S
Date:	24 March 2006
Question:	Should methadone maintenance (40–59 mg/day) versus methadone maintenance (1–39 mg/day) be used for opioid dependence?
Patient or population:	Opioid dependents
Settings:	Outpatient
Systematic review:	Faggiano F et al. *Methadone maintenance at different dosages for heroin dependence* (CLIB 3, 2003)[140].

Quality assessment						Summary of findings					
						No of patients		Effect		Quality	Importance
No. studies	Design	Limitations	Consistency	Directness	Other considerations	Methadone maintenance medium doses (40–59 mg/day)	Methadone maintenance low doses (1–39 mg/day)	Relative risk (RR) (95% CI)	Absolute risk (AR) (95% CI)		
Retention in treatment (objective follow-up: 20 weeks)											
1 a [108]	Randomized trial	No limitations b	No important inconsistency	No uncertainty	Imprecise or sparse data (−1) c	44/84 (52.4%)	34/82 (41.5%)	RR 1.26 d (0.91 to 1.75)	110/1000 more (40 less to 260 more)	⊕⊕⊕○ Moderate	7
Mortality (objective follow-up: 6 years)											
1 e [196]	Observational studies h	No limitations f	No important inconsistency	No uncertainty	Imprecise or sparse data (−1) g	1/362 (0.3%)	4/822 (0.5%)	RR 0.57 d (0.06 to 5.06)	2/1000 less (20 less to 5 more)	⊕○○○ Very low	9

a Outpatient, conducted in the United States.
b Double blind, allocation concealment unclear.
c Only one study.
d Fixed effect model.
e One CPS, outpatient, conducted in Dutch; for CPS medium doses = 55–70 mg/day, low doses = 5–55 mg/day.
f One CPS of moderate quality.
g Large confidence interval.
h CPS.

GRADE evidence profile

Author(s):	Amato L, Minozzi S
Date:	24 March 2006
Question:	Should methadone maintenance (60–120 mg/day) versus methadone maintenance (1–39 mg/day) be used for opioid dependence?
Patient or population:	Opioid dependents
Settings:	Outpatient
Systematic review:	Faggiano F et al. *Methadone maintenance at different dosages for heroin* dependence (CLIB 3, 2003)[140].

Quality assessment						Summary of findings					
						No of patients		Effect		Quality	Importance
No. studies	Design	Limitations	Consistency	Directness	Other considerations	Methadone maintenance (60–120 mg/day)	Methadone maintenance (1–39 mg/day)	Relative risk (RR) (95% CI)	Absolute risk (AR) (95% CI)		
Retention in treatment at 7–26 weeks (objective follow-up: 7–26 weeks)											
5 [141,143,205,329,330]	Randomized trials	No limitations	No important inconsistency	No uncertainty	None	138/247 (55.9%)	102/249 (41.0%)	RR 1.36 (1.13 to 1.63)	150/1000 more (50 to 260)	⊕⊕⊕⊕ High	7
Opioid abstinence (proportion of negative urine samples over 12 weeks)											
1 [330]	Randomized trials	No limitations	No important inconsistency	No uncertainty	Very imprecise or sparse data (−2)	55	55	---	WMD −2.0 (−4.8 to −0.8)	⊕⊕○○ Low	7
Opioid abstinence at 3–4 weeks (urinalysis)											
3 [141,143,205]	Randomized trials	No limitations	Inconsistent findings (−1) a	No uncertainty	Imprecise or sparse data (−1)	55/118	34/119	---	RR 1.59 (1.16 to 2.18)	⊕⊕○○ Low	7
Cocaine abstinence at 3–4 weeks (urinalysis)											
2 [143,205]	Randomized trials	No limitations	No important inconsistency	No uncertainty	Imprecise or sparse data (−1)	35/83	20/85	---	RR 1.81 (1.15 to 2.85)	⊕⊕⊕○ Moderate	6

a Significant heterogeneity.

GRADE evidence profile

Author(s):	Amato L, Minozzi S
Date:	24 March 2006
Question:	Should methadone maintenance (60–120 mg/day) versus methadone maintenance (40–59 mg/day) be used for opioid dependence?
Patient or population:	Opioid dependents
Settings:	Outpatient
Systematic review:	Faggiano F et al. *Methadone maintenance at different dosages for heroin dependence* (CLIB 3, 2003)[140].

Quality assessment						Summary of findings					
						No of patients		Effect		Quality	Importance
No. studies	Design	Limitations	Consistency	Directness	Other considerations	Methadone maintenance (60–120 mg/day)	Methadone maintenance (40–59 mg/day)	Relative risk (RR) (95% CI)	Absolute risk (AR) (95% CI)		
Retention in treatment at 7-13 weeks (Objective follow-up: 7–13 weeks)											
2[a][211, 212]	Randomized trials	No limitations[2b]	No important inconsistency	No uncertainty	Imprecise or sparse data (-1)	138/173 (79,8%)	137/174 (78,7%)	RR 1.01[c] (0.91 to 1.12)	10 more/1 000 (80 less to 90 more)	⊕⊕⊕○ Moderate	7
Retention in treatment at 27- 40 weeks (Objective follow-up: 27–40 weeks)											
3[d][211, 213, 214]	Randomized trials	No limitations[e]	No important inconsistency	No uncertainty	None	157/277 (56,7%)	130/283 (45,9%)	RR 1.23[c] (1.05 to 1.45)	100/1 000 more (30 more to 190 more)	⊕⊕⊕⊕ High	7
Opioid abstinence (Objective[g] follow-up: 3–4 weeks[j])											
1[f][212]	Randomized trials	No limitations[h]	No important inconsistency	No uncertainty	Very imprecise or sparse data (-2)[i]	10/31 (32,3%)	6/28 (21,4%)	RR 1.51[c] (0.63 to 3.61)	110/1 000 more (120 less to 330 more)	⊕⊕○○ Low	7
Criminal activity (Objective and subjective[l] Range: to . Better indicated by: lower scores)											
1[k][212]	Randomized trials	No limitations[h]	No important inconsistency	No uncertainty	Very imprecise or sparse data (-2)[i]	31	28	-	WMD 0.05 (-0.03 to 0.13)	⊕⊕○○ Low	6
Mortality (Objective follow-up: 6 years)											
1[m][196]	Observational studies[n]	No limitations[n]	No important inconsistency	No uncertainty	Very imprecise or sparse data (-2)[o]	0/316 (0%)	1/362 (0,3%)	RR 0.38[c] (0.02 to 9.34)	0/1 000 (10 less to 10 more)	⊕○○○ Very low	9

[a] Both outpatient and both conducted in USA
[b] Both double blind, allocation concealment unclear
[c] Fixed effect model
[d] All outpatient and all conducted in USA
[e] adequate allocation concealment, 2 unclear; 2 double blind, 1 single blind
[f] Outpatient, conducted in USA
[g] Based on urinalysis
[h] Double blind, allocation concealment unclear
[i] only 1 study, few participants
[j] During the treatment
[k] Outpatient, conducted in USA
[l] Medium number/week of criminal activities
[m] 1 CPS, outpatient, conducted in Dutch. For CPS high doses = >75 mg/day, medium dose = 55–70 mg/day
[n] 1 CPS of moderate quality
[o] Few events

GRADE evidence profile

Author(s):	Amato L, Minozzi S
Date:	24/03/2006
Question:	Should Methadone maintenance very high doses (>120 mg/day) versus Methadone maintenance high doses (60–120 mg/day) be used for Opioid dependence?
Patient or population:	Opioid-dependent patients Settings: Outpatient
Systematic review:	Faggiano F et al. *Methadone maintenance at different dosages for heroin dependence* (CLIB 3, 2003)[140].

Quality assessment						Summary of findings					
						No of patients		Effect		Quality	Importance
No. studies	Design	Limitations	Consistency	Directness	Other considerations	Methadone maintenance very high doses (>109 mg/day)	Methadone maintenance high doses (60-109 mg/day)	Relative risk (RR) (95% CI)	Absolute risk (AR) (95% CI)		
Retention in treatment (Objective follow-up: 27 weeks)											
1[a][213]	Randomized trials	No limitations[b]	No important inconsistency	No uncertainty	Imprecise or sparse data (-2)[c]	25/40 (62,5%)	26/40 (65%)	RR 0.96[d] (0.69 to 1.34)	30/1 000 less (240 less to 190 more)	⊕⊕○○ Low	1

[a] Outpatient, conducted in USA
[b] Single blind, adequate allocation concealment
[c] 1 study, few participants
[d] Fixed effect model

A1.6 Tapered methadone versus alpha2 adrenergic agonists for withdrawal from opioids

GRADE evidence profile

Author(s):	Amato L
Date:	02/02/2006
Question:	Should tapered methadone versus alpha2 adrenergic agonists be used in opioid users?
Patient or population:	any opioid-dependent patients wishing to withdraw from opioids
Settings:	Inpatient or outpatient
Systematic review:	Gowing L; *Alpha-2 adrenergic agonists for the management of opioid withdrawal* (CLIB 4, 2004)[222]; Amato et al.; *Methadone at tapered doses for the management of opioid withdrawal* (CLIB 3, 2005) [222].

Quality assessment						Summary of findings					
						No of patients		Effect		Quality	Importance
No. studies	Design	Limitations	Consistency	Directness	Other considerations	Tapered methadone	Alpha2 adrenergic agonists	Relative risk (RR) (95% CI)	Absolute risk (AR) (95% CI)		
completion of treatment (Objective follow-up: max 30 days[e])											
7[a] [215-221]	Randomized trials	No limitations[b]	Important inconsistency (-1)[c]	No uncertainty	None	168/251 (66,9%)	192/326 (58,9%)	RR 1.09[d] (0.90 to 1.32)	60/1 000 more (60 less to 180 more)	⊕⊕⊕○ Moderate	7
relapsed at 6 months follow-up (intention to treat (ITT) analysis) (objective follow-up: 6 months)											
1[g] [217]	Randomized trials	No limitations[h]	No important inconsistency	No uncertainty	Imprecise or sparse data (-2)[i]	11/25 (44%)	10/24 (41,7%)	RR 1.06[j] (0.55 to 2.02)	20/1 000 more (250 less to 300 more)	⊕⊕○○ Low	5

a 5/7 studies were conducted in inpatient setting, 2 in outpatient; Country of origin: USA (3), United Kingdom (2), Spain (2). There are two more studies that considered this outcome but they are observational studies, this is the reason why they have been excluded from the meta-analysis
b 2/7 studies with adequate allocation concealment, 5/7 method unclear; all double blind
c Significant heterogeneity: p = 0.0045 and no statistical significant results
d Random effect model
e Length of treatment
f The quality of reporting was very poor for this outcome. The way to report the results was very heterogeneous and prevented to pool the results in the meta-analysis. Four out of seven studies showed that alpha2 adrenergic agonists have an hypotensive effect more than methadone
g The study was conducted in USA in outpatient setting
h Double blind, unclear allocation concealment
i Only 1 study with few participants (49)
j Fixed effect model

A1.7 Medications for opioid withdrawal

GRADE evidence profile

Author(s):	Amato L
Date:	02/02/2006 16.01.56
Question:	Should tapered methadone versus tapered buprenorphine be used in all opioid-dependent patients?
Patient or population:	opioid users
Settings:	outpatient or inpatient
Systematic review:	Gowing et al.; *Buprenorphine for the management of opioid withdrawal* (CLIB 2, 2006)[159]; Amato et al.; *Methadone at tapered doses for the management of opioid withdrawal* (CLIB 3, 2005)[224].

Quality assessment						Summary of findings					
						No of patients		Effect		Quality	Importance
No. studies	Design	Limitations	Consistency	Directness	Other considerations	Tapered methadone	Tapered buprenorphine	Relative risk (RR) (95% CI)	Absolute risk (AR) (95% CI)		
Completion of treatment (Objective follow-up: 14 to 30 days[h])											
2[a][220,223]	Randomized trials	No limitations[b]	No important inconsistency	No uncertainty	Imprecise or sparse data (-2)[d]	21/30 (70%)	26/33 (78,8%)	RR 0.88[c] (0.67 to 1.15)	100/1 000 less (290 less to 100 more)	⊕⊕○○ Low	7
Side effects (variations in systolic blood pressure Range: to . Better indicated by: lower scores)											
1[e][223]	Randomized trials	No limitations[f]	No important inconsistency	No uncertainty	Imprecise or sparse data (-2)[g]	18	19	-	WMD -5.1 (-14 to 5.3)	⊕⊕○○ Low	5

[a] Both studies were conducted in inpatient setting; Country of origin: Germany (1), USA (1)
[b] 2/2 allocation concealment unclear, both double blind
[c] Random effect model
[d] Few patients (63)
[e] The study was conducted in USA with an inpatient setting
[f] Double blinded, allocation concealment unclear
[g] Only 1 study with few participants (39)
[h] Length of treatment

GRADE evidence profile

Author(s):	Amato L
Date:	13/09/2007
Question:	Should tapered buprenorphine versus alpha-2 adrenergic agonists be used for opioid withdrawal?
Patient or population:	Opiate addicts
Settings:	Outpatient and Inpatient
Systematic review:	Gowing L et al.; *Buprenorphine for the management of opioid withdrawal* (CLIB 2, 2006)[159].

Quality assessment						Summary of findings					
						No of patients		Effect		Quality	Importance
No. studies	Design	Limitations	Consistency	Directness	Other considerations	Buprenorphine	Alpha-2 adrenergic agonists	Relative risk (RR) (95% CI)	Absolute risk (AR) (95% CI)		
Completion of treatment (Objective follow-up)											
8[a][163, 225-231]	Randomized trials[b]	No limitations	Important inconsistency (-1)[f]	No uncertainty	None	317/506 (62.6%)	155/378 (41.0%)	RR 1.67[e] (1.24 to 2.25)	300/1 000 more (140 to 410)	⊕⊕⊕○ Moderate	7
Adverse effects (Objective follow-up)											
2[c][226,230]	Randomized trials[d]	No limitations	No important inconsistency	No uncertainty	None	60/292 (20,5%)	51/166 (30,7%)	RR 0.95[e] (0.77 to 1.17)	100/1 000 less (60 less to 50 more)	⊕⊕⊕⊕ High	3
Withdrawal scores (peak objective withdrawal score)											
3[c][230, 227, 231]	Randomized trials	No limitations	No important inconsistency	No uncertainty	Imprecise or sparse data (-1)	133	133	-	SMD -0.61[h] (-0.86 to -0.36)	⊕⊕⊕○ Moderate	6
Withdrawal scores (overall participant completed score)											
2[g][226, 231]	Randomized trials	No limitations	No important inconsistency	No uncertainty	None	287	165	-	SMD -0.59[g](-0.79 to -0.39)	⊕⊕⊕⊕ High	5

[a] 8 studies, 5 conducted in the USA, 1 in Australia, 1 in India and 1 in Italy
[b] For the allocation concealment, 3 rated as a, 6 b, and 1 c
[c] 3 studies, 1 conducted in Australia and 2 in USA
[d] 2 RCTs 1 rated a and 1 b
[e] random effect model
[f] significant heterogeneity
[g] 2 studies, one conducted in the US, one in Australia
[h] fixed effect model

A1.8 Should antagonists with minimal sedation be used for opioid withdrawal?

GRADE evidence profile

Author(s):	Davoli M, Amato L
Date:	02/02/2006
Question:	Should opioid antagonists with minimal sedation be used for opioid withdrawal?
Patient or population:	opioid dependents undergoing managed withdrawal
Settings:	Inpatient
Systematic review:	Gowing L et al.; *Opioid antagonists with minimal sedation for opioid with*drawal (CLIB 1, 2006)[160].

Quality assessment						Summary of findings					
						No of patients		Effect		Quality	Importance
No. studies	Design	Limitations	Consistency	Directness	Other considerations	Opioid antagonists with minimal sedation	Control	Relative risk (RR) (95% CI)	Absolute risk (AR) (95% CI)		
Completion of treatment (Objective follow-up: 3-6 days[e])											
4[a] [231-234]	Randomized trials	No limitations[b]	Important inconsistency (-1)[c]	No uncertainty	None	198/231 (85,7%)	118/163 (72,4%)	RR 1.26[d] (0.80 to 2.00)	70/1 000 (40 less to 180 more)	⊕⊕⊕○ Moderate	7
Severity and duration of withdrawal symptoms (Subjective and objective follow-up)											
4[a] [231, 235-237]	Randomized trials	Serious limitations (-1)[b, f]	No important inconsistency[g]	No uncertainty	High probability of reporting bias (-1)[g]	-	-	Unable to compare scales	-	⊕⊕○○ Low	5
Side effects (Subjective follow-up: 3-6 days[e])											
2[h] [235, 237]	Observational studies[n]	No limitations[i]	No important inconsistency	No uncertainty	Imprecise or sparse data (-1)[f] High probability of reporting bias (-1)[f, j]	6/94 (6,4%)	1/80 (1,2%)	RR 3.71[d] (0.65 to 21.32)	50/1 000 more (10 less to 110 more)	⊕○○○ Very low	8
Patients who have relapsed at follow-up (Subjective follow-up: 6 months)											
1[k] [234]	Randomized trials	No limitations[l]	No important inconsistency	Some uncertainty (-1)[m]	Imprecise or sparse data (-1)[m]	15/32 (46,9%)	18/32 (56,2%)	RR 0.83 (0.52 to 1.35)	100/1 000 less (2700 less to 100 more)	⊕⊕○○ Low	5

a Country of origin of the studies: Italy (2), United Kingdom (1) and USA (1); 3 studies were conducted in an outpatient setting, 1 inpatient
b 3/4 the allocation concealment was unclear, and in 1/4 inadequate; 2 double blind, 2 no information on blindness
c Statistically significant heterogeneity
d Random effect model
e Length of treatment
f In addition, there are major differences in treatment schedules and the type of additional therapy
g Measured on the basis of subjective symptoms using different scales preventing the possibility of pooling data
h 2 controlled prospective trial, both conducted in USA and in outpatient setting
i Allocation concealment unclear in 1 study and inadequate in the other
j The RR is greater than 3
k The study was conducted in Italy in outpatient setting
l Unclear allocation concealment, no information on blindness
m only 1 study, few participants (98) and conducted in outpatient setting
n Observational studies

A1.9 Should opioid antagonists with heavy sedation or anaesthesia be used for opioid withdrawal?

GRADE evidence profile

Author(s):	Davoli M, Amato L
Date:	02/02/2006
Question:	Should opioid antagonist under heavy sedation be used for opioid withdrawal?
Patient or population:	opioid-dependent patients undergoing managed withdrawal
Settings:	Inpatient
Systematic review:	Gowing L et al.; *Opioid antagonists under heavy sedation or anaesthesia for opioid withdrawal* (CLIB 2, 2006)[161].

Quality assessment						Summary of findings					
						No of patients		Effect		Quality	Importance
No. studies	Design	Limitations	Consistency	Directness	Other considerations	Opioid antagonist under heavy sedation	Standard opioid withdrawal	Relative risk (RR) (95% CI)	Absolute risk (AR) (95% CI)		
Completion of treatment[e] (clonidine comparison) (Objective follow-up: 1-3 days[d])											
2[a][162,163]	Randomized trials	No limitations[b]	No important inconsistency	No uncertainty	Imprecise or sparse data (-1)	74/86 (86%)	95/121 (78,5%)	RR 1.15[c] (0.79 to 1.68)	150/1 000 more (140 less to 350 more)	⊕⊕⊕○ Moderate	7
Completion of treatment[e] (buprenorphine comparison) (Objective follow-up: 1-3 days[d])											
1[163]	Randomized trials	No limitations[b]	No important inconsistency	No uncertainty	Imprecise or sparse data (-2)	7/35 (20%)	9/37 (24,3%)	RR 0.82[c] (0.34 to 1.97)	50 less/1 000 (230less to 150 more)	⊕⊕○○ Low	7
Commencement of naltrexone (clonidine comparison)											
2[162,163]	Randomized trials	No limitations	No important inconsistency	No uncertainty	Imprecise or sparse data (-1)	73/86 (85%)	21/84 (25%)	RR 3.4[c] (2.32 to 4.98)		⊕⊕⊕○ Moderate	5
Commencement of naltrexone (buprenorphine comparison)											
1[163]	Randomized trials	No limitations	No important inconsistency	No uncertainty	Imprecise or sparse data (-2)	33/35 (94%)	36/37 (97%)	RR 0.97[c] (0.88 to 1.07)		⊕⊕○○ Low	5
Severity and duration of withdrawal (subjective rating scales follow-up:)											
1[f][163]	Randomized trials	No limitations[g]	No important inconsistency	No uncertainty	Imprecise or sparse data (-1)[h] High probability of reporting bias (-1)[i]	/	/	unable to compare scales	-	⊕⊕○○ Low	7
Adverse events (Objective follow-up: 1-4 days[d])											
2[162,163]	Randomized trials	No limitations	No important inconsistency	No uncertainty	Imprecise or sparse data (-1)	14/287 (5%)	4/285 (1.4%)	RR 3.41 (1.13 to 9.12)		⊕⊕⊕○ Moderate	6
Life threatening adverse events (Objective follow-up: 1-4 days[d])											
1[f][163]	Randomized trials	No limitations[g]	No important inconsistency	No uncertainty	Imprecise or sparse data (-2)[j]	3/35 (8,6%)	0/71 (0%)	RR 14[c] (0.74 to 263.78)	90/1 000 (10 less to 180 more)	⊕⊕○○ Low	9
Relapsed at follow-up (ITT analysis) (Objective (urine analysis) follow-up: 12 months)											
2[a][162,163]	Randomized trials	No limitations[b]	No important inconsistency	No uncertainty[m]	Imprecise or sparse data (-1)	74/86 (86%)	109/121 (90,1%)	RR 0.97[3] (0.88 to 1.08)	30/1 000 less (110 less to 70 more)	⊕⊕⊕○ Moderate	5
Retention at 12 months (Objective follow-up: 12 months)											
2[a][162,163]	Randomized trials	No limitations[b]	No important inconsistency	No uncertainty	Imprecise or sparse data (-1)	35/86 (40,7%)	43/121 (35,5%)	RR 0.95[c] (0.69 to 1.30)	20/1 000 less (110 less to 110 more)	⊕⊕⊕○ Moderate	5

[a] The countries in which the 2 studies were conducted are: USA (1), Australia (1), both trials were conducted with inpatients.
[b] In both studies method of allocation concealment was not stated, 1 study was single blind (patients blind) and the other one no blindness
[c] Fixed effect model
[d] Length of treatment
[e] The outcome is not relevant in this context
[f] The study was conducted in the USA in inpatient setting
[g] Method of allocation concealment not stated, no blindness
[h] Only one study and data based on self-reporting
[i] Based on self-reporting and no dose response effect shown by other 2 RCTs for withdrawal symptoms and duration
[j] Only one study and few participants (106)
[k] This is a relevant outcome
[l] Dose response effect shown by other 2 RCTs comparing different doses
[m] Data based on study with very high proportion of patients lost to follow-up
[n] Only two studies, few participants (78)

A1.10 Should withdrawal from opioids be conducted in inpatient or outpatient settings?

GRADE evidence profile

Author(s):	Amato L
Date:	02/02/2006
Question:	Should inpatient detoxification treatment versus outpatient detoxification treatment be used for opioid detoxification?
Patient or population:	opioid users
Settings:	inpatient versus outpatient
Systematic review:	Day E. et al.; *Inpatient versus other settings for detoxification for opioid dependence* (CLIB 2, 2005)[168].

Quality assessment						Summary of findings				Quality	Importance
						No of patients		Effect			
No. studies	Design	Limitations	Consistency	Directness	Other considerations	Inpatient detoxification treatment	Outpatient detoxification treatment	Relative risk (RR) (95% CI)	Absolute risk (AR) (95% CI)		
Completion of treatment (objective follow-up: 10 days[d])											
1[a] [238]	Randomized trials	Serious limitations (-1)[b]	No important inconsistency	No uncertainty	Imprecise or sparse data (-2)[e]	7/10 (70%)	11/30 (36,7%)	RR 1.91[c] (1.03 to 3.55)	330/1 000 more (0 to 670 more)	⊕○○○ Very low	7
Relapsed at follow-up (Objective follow-up: 10 days)											
1[a] [238]	Randomized trials	Serious limitations (-1)[b]	No important inconsistency	No uncertainty	Imprecise or sparse data (-2)[e]	10/10 (100%)	28/30 (93,3%)	RR 1.07[c] (0.97 to 1.18)	70/1 000 more (90 less to 220 more)	⊕○○○ Very low	7

[a] The study was conducted in USA
[b] There are serious methodological problems regarding the randomization method
[c] Fixed effect model
[d] Length of treatment
[e] Very few participants (40)

A1.11 Should antagonist pharmacotherapy, naltrexone, be used for the treatment of opioid dependence?

GRADE evidence profile

Author(s):	Minozzi S, Amato L
Date:	23/03/2006
Question:	Should oral naltrexone be used for opioid dependence?
Patient or population:	Opioid-dependent patients
Settings:	Outpatient
Systematic review:	Minozzi et al.; *Oral naltrexone treatment for opioid dependence* (CLIB 1, 2006)[170].

Quality assessment						Summary of findings				Quality	Importance
						No of patients		Effect			
No. studies	Design	Limitations	Consistency	Directness	Other considerations	Oral naltrexone	Placebo	Relative risk (RR) (95% CI)	Absolute risk (AR) (95% CI)		
Retention in treatment (Objective follow-up: 2-9 months[d])											
5[a] [239-243]	Randomized trials	No limitations[b]	No important inconsistency	No uncertainty	Imprecise or sparse data (-1)	35/105 (33,3%)	31/98 (31,6%)	RR 1.08[c] (0.74 to 1.57)	20/1 000 more (90 less to 140 more)	⊕⊕⊕○ Moderate	6
Use of opioids (Objective[f] follow-up: 2-9 months[d])											
6[e] [239-244]	Randomized trials	Serious limitations (-1)[g]	No important inconsistency	No uncertainty	Imprecise or sparse data (-1)	68/139 (48,9%)	69/110 (62,7%)	RR 0.72[c] (0.58 to 0.90)	180 less / 1 000 (290 less to 60 less)	⊕⊕○○ Low	7
Relapsed at follow-up (follow-up: 6 months-1 year)											
2[h] [241, 242]	Randomized trials	No limitations[i]	No important inconsistency	No uncertainty	Imprecise or sparse data (-2)[j]	26/43 (60,5%)	24/38 (63,2%)	RR 0.94[c] (0.67 to 1.34)	40 less / 1 000 (250 less to 180 more)	⊕⊕○○ Low	7
Criminal behaviour (objective[o] follow-up: 6-10 months[d])											
2[n] [245, 246]	Randomized trials	No limitations[p]	No important inconsistency	Specific population (prison release) (-1)	Imprecise or sparse data (-2)	13/54 (24,1%)	15/32 (46,9%)	RR 0.50[c] (0.27 to 0.91)	240 less / 1 000 (440 less to 30 less)	⊕○○○ Very low	6

[a] Outpatient. Country of origin: Israel 2, USA 1, Russia 1, Spain 1
[b] 2 adequate allocation concealment, the other unclear; all double blind
[c] Fixed effect model
[d] Length of treatment
[e] All outpatient. Country of origin: Israel 2, USA 1, China 1, Russia 1, Spain 1
[f] Based on urinalysis
[g] 2 adequate allocation concealment, the other unclear; all double blind. ITT analyses not used.
[h] Both outpatient, one conducted in Israel, the other in Spain
[i] 1 with adequate allocation concealment, 1 unclear, both double blind
[j] Few patients, result not statistically significant
[k] All outpatient, conducted in USA, China and Russia 1 each
[l] 1 adequate allocation concealment, 2 unclear, all double blind
[m] Number of subjects with at least one side effect
[n] Both outpatient and both conducted in USA
[o] Number re-incarcerated
[p] Both unclear allocation concealment and open design
[q] 2 studies, few patients

A1.12 Should psychosocial treatments be used in addition to pharmacological maintenance treatments?

GRADE evidence profile

Author(s):	Amato L, Minozzi S
Date:	23/03/2006
Question:	Should psychosocial plus pharmacological maintenance treatments versus pharmacological maintenance treatments alone be used for opioid dependence?
Patient or population:	Opiate dependent patients
Settings:	Outpatient
Systematic review:	Amato et al.; *Psychosocial combined with agonist maintenance treatments versus agonist maintenance treatments alone for treatment of opioid dependence* (CLIB 4, 2004)[257].

Quality assessment						Summary of findings					
						No of patients		Effect		Quality	Importance
No. studies	Design	Limitations	Consistency	Directness	Other considerations	Psychosocial plus pharmacological maintenance treatments	Pharmacological maintenance treatments alone	Relative risk (RR) (95% CI)	Absolute risk (AR) (95% CI)		
Retention in treatment (Objective follow-up: 6-24 weeks[d])											
8[a] [212, 247-253]	Randomized trials	No limitations[b]	No important inconsistency	No uncertainty	None	228/296 (77%)	170/214 (79,4%)	RR 0.94[c,e] (0.85 to 1.02)	50 less / 1 000 (120 less to 20 more)	⊕⊕⊕⊕ High	7
Use of opioids (Objective[g] follow-up: 6-32 weeks[d])											
5[f] [156, 251-254]	Randomized trials	No limitations[h]	No important inconsistency	No uncertainty	None	70/187 (37,4%)	105/201 (52,2%)	RR 0.69[j] (0.53 to 0.91)	190 less / 1 000 (320 less to 50 less)	⊕⊕⊕⊕ High	7
Retention in treatment at the end of follow-up (Objective follow-up: 4-48 weeks)											
3[i] [248, 255, 256]	Randomized trials	No limitations[k]	No important inconsistency	No uncertainty	None	105/163 (64,4%)	62/87 (71,3%)	RR 0.90[c] (0.76 to 1.07)	70 less / 1 000 (190 less to 50 more)	⊕⊕⊕⊕ High	7
Abstinent at the end of follow-up (follow-up: 1-12 months)											
2[l] [248, 256]	Randomized trials	No limitations[m]	Important inconsistency (-1)[n]	No uncertainty	Imprecise or sparse data (-1)[n]	44/70 (62,9%)	27/38 (71,1%)	RR 0.88[c] (0.67 to 1.15)	90 less / 1 000 (260 less to 90 more)	⊕⊕○○ Low	6

[a] All outpatient and all conducted in USA
[b] All but 1 unclear allocation concealment, 1 inadequate; 2 double blind
[c] Fixed effect model
[d] Length of treatment
[e] Excluding the study with inadequate allocation concealment the result do not change
[f] All outpatient and all conducted in USA
[g] Based on urinalysis
[h] All with unclear allocation concealment, 1 double blind
[i] Random effect model
[j] All outpatient and all conducted in USA
[k] All with unclear allocation concealment, 1 double blind
[l] Both outpatient and both conducted in USA
[m] 1 double blind, 2 unclear allocation concealment
[n] Two studies with conflicting results

A1.13 Is psychosocial assistance plus pharmacological assistance for opioid withdrawal more useful than pharmacological assistance alone?

GRADE evidence profile

Author(s):	Hill S, Davoli M, Amato L
Date:	02/02/2006
Question:	Should any pharmacological withdrawal treatment plus psychosocial treatment versus any pharmacological withdrawal treatment alone be used in opioid-dependent patients requiring withdrawal?
Patient or population:	Opioid users
Settings:	Outpatients
Systematic review:	Amato et al.; *Psychosocial and pharmacological treatments versus pharmacological treatments for opioid detoxification* (CLIB 2, 2004)[169].

Quality assessment						Summary of findings				Quality	Importance
						No of patients		Effect			
No. studies	Design	Limitations	Consistency	Directness	Other considerations	Pharmacological withdrawal plus psychosocial treatment	Pharmacological withdrawal alone	Relative risk (RR) (95% CI)	Absolute risk (AR) (95% CI)		
Completion of treatment (Objective follow-up: average 18 weeks, range 2-52[e])											
5[a][258-262]	Randomized trials	No limitations[b]	No important inconsistency	No uncertainty	Imprecise or sparse data (-1)	37/89 (41,6%)	24/95 (25,3%)	RR 1.68[c,e] (1.11 to 2.55)	170 more / 1 000 (40 more to 300 more)	⊕⊕⊕○ Moderate	7
Use of primary substance during treatment (urine samples) (follow-up: average 18 weeks, range 2-52[d])											
3[a][258, 260, 261]	Randomized trials	No limitations[f]	No important inconsistency	No uncertainty	Imprecise or sparse data (-1)[g]	40/55 (72.7%)	30/54 (55.6%)	RR 1.30[c] (0.99 to 1.70)	170 more / 1 000 (10 less to 330 more)	⊕⊕⊕○ Moderate	7
Relapsed at follow-up (Objective: urine test. follow-up: 1 year)											
3[a][258, 261, 263]	Randomized trials	No limitations[f]	No important inconsistency	No uncertainty	Imprecise or sparse data (-1)	25/123 (20.3%)	38/85 (44.7%)	RR 0.41[c,m] (0.27 to 0.62)	280 less / 1 000 (400 less to 150 less)	⊕⊕⊕○ Moderate	7
Subjects using other substances: barbiturates (Objective: urine samples) follow-up: 16 weeks[e])											
1[h][258]	Randomized trials	No limitations[i]	No important inconsistency	No uncertainty	Very imprecise or sparse data (-2)[j]	9/19 (47,4%)	6/20 (30%)	RR 1.58[c] (0.70 to 3.59)	170 more / 1 000 (130 less to 470 more)	⊕○○○ Very low	4
Subjects using other substances: benzodiazepines (Objective (urine samples) follow-up: 16 weeks[e])											
1[h][258]	Randomized trials	No limitations[i]	No important inconsistency	No uncertainty	Very imprecise or sparse data (-2)[l]	15/19 (75%)	17/20 (89.5%)	RR 0.84[c] (0.62 to 1.13)	140 less / 1 000 (380 less to 90 more)	⊕○○○ Very low	4
Subjects using other substances: cocaine (urine test follow-up: 16 weeks[e])											
1[h][258]	Randomized trials	No limitations[i]	No important inconsistency	No uncertainty	Very imprecise or sparse data (-2)[l]	11/19 (55%)	12/20 (63.2%)	RR 0.87[c] (0.52 to 1.47)	80 less / 1 000 (390 less to 230 more)	⊕○○○ Very low	5

[a] All studies were conducted in the USA and all in outpatient setting
[b] Four studies with unclear allocation concealment and one with inadequate; 2 studies were single blind (participants blind only for pharmacological interventions) and 3 did not report data on blindness
[c] Fixed effect model
[d] Performing a sensitivity analysis excluding the study with inadequate allocation concealment (class C) from meta-analysis (Robles 2002, 48 participants)[262]. The result did not change, remaining significantly in favour of the associated treatments (RR 0.46 (95% CI 0.27 to 0.79)
[e] Length of treatment
[f] All studies with unclear allocation concealment, 2 single blind an 1 not blind
[g] Few patients (109)
[h] The study was conducted in USA, in outpatient setting (Bickel 1997)[258]
[i] Unclear allocation concealment, single blind
[j] Only one study, few participants and wide confidence interval
[k] Low generalizability of treatments offered
[l] Only one study, few participants
[m] Performing a sensitivity analysis excluding the study with inadequate allocation concealment (class C) from meta-analysis (Yandoli 2002, 119 participants)[263]. The result became not statistically significant RR 0.84 (95% CI 0.68 to 1.04)
[n] Inadequate allocation concealment, open label
[o] Few patients and wide confidence interval
[p] The study was conducted in USA, in an outpatient setting (Yandoli, 2002)[263]

Annex 2 Dispensing, dosing and prescriptions

A2.1 Dispensing

Dispensing of methadone and buprenorphine may take place in a variety of clinical and community settings.

In specialist clinical settings, an onsite pharmacy or dispensary can enable observation of patients at the time of each dosing. This observation means that clinic staff can more thoroughly assess patients whom they would normally observe less frequently. In community settings, dispensing may occur at community pharmacies or, in some countries, buprenorphine may be dispensed in a physician's office.

Dispensing staff can make a valuable contribution to multidisciplinary care planning, which is more easily accommodated in the clinic setting. In the community setting, where agonist treatment is dispensed in community pharmacies, medical staff should be encouraged to discuss patients regularly with the dispensing pharmacist, to determine, if applicable, the number of missed doses or the level of intoxication on presentation for dosing. If the pharmacy that is dispensing the methadone or buprenorphine is external to the agency prescribing the methadone or buprenorphine, then patients should be informed, before they commence methadone or buprenorphine, that communication with the external pharmacy is a condition of treatment.

Methadone and buprenorphine should be kept in a secure safe, according to local requirements. The amounts should be checked and witnessed by a second party daily, to ensure the amount used is reconciled with amount dispensed.

Generally, dispensing staff are pharmacists, although in most jurisdictions, medical and nursing staff can also dispense medication. Pharmacists and other dispensing staff should be trained in the issues involved in dispensing methadone and buprenorphine.

Before dispensing methadone and buprenorphine, dispensing staff should:
- establish the identity of the patient and confirm this with the name on the prescription
- confirm that the patient is not intoxicated
- check that the prescription is valid and that the current day is a dosing day (for alternate days or three-times-a-week buprenorphine prescriptions)
- confirm the dose of the prescription.

To further reduce dosing errors and assist with record keeping, computerized systems are available that confirm the identity of the patient using retinal or iris scanners, and automatically dispense the dose on the prescription (after it has been entered by the pharmacist).

It is vital that methadone or buprenorphine are not dispensed to people who are sedated or intoxicated because this may lead to over sedation. Dispensing staff should be skilled in the assessment of the degree of sedation and confident in refusing doses to intoxicated patients. It can be helpful to test breath alcohol levels if patients have been drinking. Patients who present intoxicated or sedated should be asked to return when the intoxication or sedation has abated.

The dose dispensed should be recorded in accordance with jurisdictional requirements.

A2.2 Administration of buprenorphine

Buprenorphine tablets should be dispensed in a dry dosing cup after the number and strength of the tablets have been checked. Before administration, a patient should be advised to place the tablets under the tongue and to refrain from swallowing (tablets or saliva) until the tablets have dissolved (5 minutes on average , but can take up to 15 minutes). The pharmacist should check a patient's mouth cavity for food or receptacles that might be used to divert buprenorphine. After administration, the pharmacist should check the patient's mouth cavity again, to determine that the buprenorphine has dissolved. The patient should then be offered a drink to rinse the mouth cavity.

To avoid disputes over doses, patients should indicate that they have received a dose in some way, such as by signing a dosing card. If a patient attempts to spit out a dose or to leave the dispensary before the dose has dissolved, the prescribing doctor should be informed. Crushing buprenorphine tablets into course granules has been tried in some places to limit diversion of buprenorphine, but the efficacy of this approach has not been evaluated.

A2.3 Prescriptions

Legal requirements for prescriptions vary by jurisdiction; however, in general a prescription for opioid agonist maintenance therapy should specify the following:
- name, address and telephone number of the prescribing doctor
- name of the pharmacy to dispense methadone or buprenorphinename and address of the patient
- date of the prescription
- preparation to be dispensed (i.e. methadone liquid or buprenorphine sublingual tablets)
- dose to be dispensed in milligrams (words and numbers)
- frequency of dispensing (daily, twice daily, alternate daily, three times a week)
- start and end dates of dosing covered by the prescription
- whether doses are to be supervised or if some are to be taken away (specify the maximum number that can be taken home per week)..

Because of the potential seriousness of dosing error, some jurisdictions ensure that the prescribing medical practitioner endorses a photograph of the patient, which is supplied to the pharmacy or dispensing point. It is a requirement in some jurisdictions for doses of opioids to be written in both words and figures. To reduce prescription fraud, it can be useful to send a copy of the prescription to the pharmacy by facsimile or secure email.

Annex 3 ICD-10 codes for conditions covered in these guidelines

This annex describes the codes from the *International Classification of Diseases*, 10th edition (ICD-10) that are relevant to these guidelines[14].

F11.0 Intoxication (opioids)

A condition that follows the administration of a psychoactive substance resulting in disturbances in level of consciousness, cognition, perception, affect or behaviour, or other psycho-physiological functions and responses. The disturbances are directly related to the acute pharmacological effects of the substance and resolve with time, with complete recovery, except where tissue damage or other complications have arisen. Complications may include trauma, inhalation of vomitus, delirium, coma, convulsions, and other medical complications. The nature of these complications depends on the pharmacological class of substance and mode of administration.

Excludes: intoxication meaning poisoning (T36–T50).

F11.2 Dependence syndrome (opioids)

A cluster of behavioural, cognitive, and physiological phenomena that develop after repeated substance use and that typically include a strong desire to take the drug, difficulties in controlling its use, persisting in its use despite harmful consequences, a higher priority given to drug use than to other activities and obligations, increased tolerance, and sometimes a physical withdrawal state.

The dependence syndrome may be present for a specific psychoactive substance (e.g. tobacco, alcohol, or diazepam), for a class of substances (e.g. opioid drugs), or for a wider range of pharmacologically different psychoactive substances.

The ICD-10 diagnostic criteria for opioid dependence are:
- a strong desire or sense of compulsion to take opioids
- difficulties in controlling opioid-use behaviours in terms of the onset, termination or levels of use
- a physiological withdrawal state when opioid use has ceased or been reduced, as evidenced by one of the following:
  - the characteristic withdrawal syndrome
  - use of opioids (or closely related substances) with the intention of relieving or avoiding withdrawal symptoms
- evidence of tolerance, such that increased doses of opioids are required to achieve effects originally produced by lower doses
- progressive neglect of alternative pleasures or interests because of opioid use; increased amounts of time spent to obtain opioids or to recover from their effects
- persisting with opioid use despite clear evidence of overtly harmful consequences, such as depressive mood states consequent to periods of heavy substance use, or drug-related impairment of cognitive functioning (efforts should be made to determine that the user was actually, or could be expected to be, aware of the nature and extent of the harm).

Narrowing of the personal repertoire of patterns of opioid use has also been described as a characteristic feature of dependence.

Opioid dependence does not develop without a period of regular use, although regular use alone is not sufficient to induce dependence.

A definite diagnosis of dependence should usually be made only if three or more of the diagnostic criteria have been experienced or exhibited concurrently at some time during the previous 12 months.

F11.3 Withdrawal state (opioids)

A group of symptoms of variable clustering and severity occurring on absolute or relative withdrawal of a psychoactive substance after persistent use of that substance. The onset and course of the withdrawal state are time-limited and are related to the type of psychoactive substance and dose being used immediately before cessation or reduction of use. The withdrawal state may be complicated by convulsions.

Annex 4 Pharmacology of medicines available for the treatment of opioid dependence

A4.1 Methadone

Methadone is a potent synthetic opioid agonist. It has two oral formulations, a tablet and a solution. The solution is recommended for the treatment of opioid dependence because it is easier to supervise the consumption of a liquid than a tablet and because take-home doses can be diluted to reduce the risk of injection. Both oral formulations have a bitter taste.

In opioid-naive people, the effects of methadone are qualitatively similar to morphine and other opiates; however, in opioid-dependent people, methadone prevents withdrawal symptoms without producing significant sedation or intoxication.

Methadone has a high (85%) oral bioavailability (i.e. the proportion of a therapeutically active drug that reaches the systemic circulation and is available at the site of action after being consumed orally). Peak plasma concentrations are generally 2–4 hours after dosing. Methadone is distributed widely in tissues and protein binding is reported to be 60 to 90%. Methadone is demethylated via hepatic cytochrome P450 3A4 (CYP3A4) and 2D6 (CYP2D6) enzymes to its major metabolite 2-ethylidine-1,5-dimethyl-3,3-diphenylpyrrolidine (EDDP). This inactive metabolite is excreted in the faeces and urine, together with unchanged methadone. Concomitant use of drugs that affect these enzymes may result in clinically significant interactions. Methadone doses should be adjusted accordingly.

Declining plasma concentrations have been reported during methadone maintenance, suggesting that tolerance occurs, possibly as a result of autoinduction of hepatic microsomal enzymes.

Marked inter-individual variations in absorption, distribution, circulation, metabolism or elimination (kinetics) have been observed with methadone. Elimination half-lives vary considerably – a range of 15 to 60 hours has been reported – and careful adjustment of dosage is necessary with repeated administration, after which there is a gradual accumulation in the tissues.

Methadone is included in Schedule I of the Single Convention in Narcotic Drugs, 1961 (see Annex 7).

A4.2 Buprenorphine

Buprenorphine is a potent synthetic partial opioid agonist with high receptor affinity and slow receptor dissociation. This means that its clinical effects vary both on the level of neuroadaptation of the person consuming the buprenorphine (tolerance) and the level of receptor occupancy at the time of its use (the timing of most recent opioid use). The partial activity of buprenorphine means that it does not induce tolerance to opioids to the same extent as methadone. Its high receptor affinity means that buprenorphine can block the effects of additional opioid use without inducing the same degree of tolerance as methadone. Its slow receptor dissociation and partial activity combined mean that it has a withdrawal syndrome that is milder that methadone.

Under low levels of opioid neuroadaptation, all doses of buprenorphine produce agonist effects, with high doses producing qualitatively similar effects to low doses, but for a longer period of time. However, under high levels of neuroadaptation with recent opioid use, high doses of buprenorphine can displace heroin and other opioids from receptors, leading to a rapid drop in opioid effect, which is experienced as opioid withdrawal.

Low doses of buprenorphine have been used extensively in many countries for the management of acute pain.

The potential advantage of buprenorphine is that it has a very good margin of safety. Its partial agonist activity at the μ opioid receptor prevents buprenorphine from causing the potentially fatal respiratory depression that is associated with excessive ingestion of full agonist opioids. This margin of safety also allows higher doses to be used for the purposes of prolonging action, without significantly increasing the opioid effect. In this way a double dose of buprenorphine can be given every second day, with no dose in between.

Buprenorphine is included in Schedule III of the Convention on Psychotropic Substances, 1971.

A4.3 Buprenorphine–naloxone 4:1 combination product

A combination product of buprenorphine and naloxone in a 4:1 ratio is available in two-dose strengths (2 mg buprenorphine:0.5 mg naloxone and 8 mg buprenorphine:2 mg naloxone). The efficacy of this medication is not reviewed in these guidelines due to the lack of clinical trials; however, as this drug is registered and used in several countries, the pharmacology is reviewed here.

While buprenorphine is absorbed sublingually, naloxone has only a 5–10% sublingual absorption[267]. It is thought that this results in too low a dose to have an effect clinically. As buprenorphine and naloxone have similar affinity for opioid receptors, the buprenorphine effect dominates because it is present in much higher concentrations in the blood. However, if the buprenorphine/naloxone combination product is injected, the dose of naloxone can induce opioid withdrawal, depending on the circumstances.

In the dependent user of heroin or other opioid agonists, the injection of the buprenorphine–naloxone combination product results in opioid withdrawal[268, 269]. Higher doses of buprenorphine–naloxone induce more significant withdrawal[270]. In the non-dependent opioid user, injection of the buprenorphine–naloxone product does not induce opioid withdrawal, but the opioid effect of buprenorphine is attenuated by the naloxone, resulting in a delayed and reduced opioid effect[271]. For patients in treatment using buprenorphine, or for those using buprenorphine illicitly, injection of the buprenorphine–naloxone product does not appear to induce withdrawal[272], either because higher doses of naloxone are needed to displace buprenorphine or because the half-life of naloxone is too short in comparison with the slow dissociation of buprenorphine from opioid receptors.

A4.4 Opioid antagonist medications

Naltrexone

Naltrexone is an orally active opioid antagonist, with an effective duration of action of 24–48 hours, making it suitable for use once a day. It has a very high affinity for opioid receptors and will displace heroin and methadone in minutes, and buprenorphine in 1–4 hours. It is used clinically after opioid withdrawal to prevent relapse to opioid dependence.

Naloxone

Naloxone is a short-acting injectable opioid antagonist used in the management of opioid overdose to reverse the effects of opioids. It is poorly absorbed orally and so is used either intramuscularly or intravenously. It has a half-life of approximately one hour but continues to have 50% receptor occupancy at 2 hours after injection due to its receptor binding [273].

A4.5 Medication for the management of opioid withdrawal

Alpha adrenergic agonists

The alpha-2 agonists clonidine, lofexidine and guanfacine act on the central and peripheral autonomic nervous system, reducing the endogenous release of adrenaline and noradrenalin, which are in comparative excess in opioid withdrawal. This slows the heart rate, lowers blood pressure, reduces muscle tone and induces sedation. Lofexidine is more specific to peripheral actions and does not induce hypotension to the same extent. Both lofexidine and clonidine are short acting and are taken four times a day. Guanfacine, on the other hand, is taken once a day.

Annex 5 Drug interactions involving methadone and buprenorphine

Drug interactions occur because medications have synergistic or antagonistic effects (so-called pharmacodynamic interactions), or because the presence of one medication affects the absorption, distribution, circulation, metabolism or elimination of another medication (so-called pharmacokinetic interactions).

A5.1 Pharmacodynamic interactions

Sedation

Any drugs that cause sedation may cause additive sedation with methadone and buprenorphine, increasing the risk of sedative overdose. Such drugs include benzodiazepines, alcohol, other sedative psychotropic medications (e.g. phenothiazines and other antipsychotics), tricyclic and other sedating antidepressants, alpha adrenergic agonists (e.g. clonidine and lofexidine) and sedative antihistamines. Most overdose deaths associated with methadone and buprenorphine are in combination with one or more of these sedatives.

Opioid withdrawal

Opiate antagonists, such as naltrexone, result in opioid withdrawal for patients on methadone and buprenorphine. Naltrexone cannot be used for the management of alcohol dependence in this population. A combination of agonists and partial agonists can also result in opioid withdrawal. Methadone should generally not be combined with the partial agonists buprenorphine, pentazocine, nalbuphine or butorphanol. Patients on buprenorphine who are also taking opioid agonists for pain may experience incomplete pain relief.

QT prolongation

A group of medications affect the time it takes cardiac ventricular muscle to depolarize and subsequently repolarize – the QT interval in an electrocardiogram. A prolongation of the QT interval predisposes people to serious cardiac arrhythmias, such as *torsades de pointes* and other ventricular tachyarrhythmias, which may be fatal if untreated. Methadone is one such medication. Combinations of methadone with other medications that prolong the QT interval should be used with caution, as they may further increase the risk of QT prolongation-associated cardiac arrhythmias. These medications are mainly class I or III antiarrhythmic agents, calcium channel blocking agents, some antipsychotic agents and some antidepressants (see Table A5.1 for a more complete list). Drugs that result in electrolyte disorders (e.g. hypokalaemia and hypomagnesaemia) also result in an increased risk of QT prolongation-related arrhythmias (i.e. diuretics, laxatives, corticosteroid hormones with mineralocorticoid activity). Buprenorphine does not appear to produce clinically significant prolongation of the QT interval.

A5.2 Pharmacokinetic interactions

Methadone and buprenorphine are metabolized principally by the cytochrome P450 enzyme pathways. A range of drugs and medication either induce or inhibit cytochrome P450 enzymes. The process of induction is relatively slow as it depends on the synthesis of new enzyme proteins, and occurs over days, whereas inhibition can occur rapidly, depending on the concentration of the inhibiting substance.

Methadone is largely metabolized from active to largely inactive metabolites through CYP3A4 and to a lesser extent CYP1A2, CYP2D6, CYP2B6, CYP2C8 and also possibly CYP2C9 and CYP2C19[275, 276, 277, 278, 279, 280, 281, 282, 283]. CYP enzyme inducers can result in lower plasma methadone levels and inhibitors can result in higher levels. Because of the potential for sedative overdose, patients on methadone should be observed particularly closely when commencing cytochrome P450 inhibitors, and consideration should be given to simultaneous methadone reduction. After introducing a potentially interacting new medicine, it is important to make careful clinical observations and adjust the dose of methadone if necessary.

Buprenorphine is metabolized in the liver, principally by the CYP3A4 isoenzyme[282]. The active metabolite, nor-buprenorphine is metabolized via a separate pathway. Drugs that inhibit CYP3A4 (e.g. ketoconazole, erythromycin, some protease inhibitors) may result in increases in buprenorphine concentration and the need to reduce the buprenorphine dose. Drugs that induce CYP3A4 (e.g. rifampicin, phenytoin, phenobarbital, carbamazepine) may result in reduced buprenorphine concentrations. Research on drug interactions involving buprenorphine is limited.

A more comprehensive list of drugs that interact on the cytochrome P450 system are listed in Table A5.2[282].

CYP450 inducers

Alcohol
Chronic consumption of alcohol has been reported to increase the metabolism of methadone, whereas acute consumption has been reported to increase the area under the curve (AUC)[1] of methadone, resulting in increased potential for adverse effects.

Anticonvulsants
Phenytoin, carbamazepine and phenobarbital are all significant inducers of CYP3A4 and have all resulted in withdrawal symptoms in patients on methadone.

Antidepressants
Sertraline, fluoxetine and fluvoxamine are inducers of CYP3A4. Methadone may potentiate the effects of tricyclic antidepressants.

Antimycobacterials
Rifampicin (rifampin) has resulted in clinically significant reductions in methadone levels.

---

1 Area under the curve is a measure of the bioavailability of a drug or medicine. It is the area under the plasma concentration-time curve for that drug in a particular patient. Increase in this indicates more of the drug has reached the systemic circulation and this is nearly always accompanied by a rise in plasma concentration.

Table A5.1 Drugs that increase the risk of torsades de pointes or QT interval prolongation			
Amiodarone	Arsenic trioxide	Bepridil	Chloroquine
Chlorpromazine	Cisapride	Clarithromycin	Disopyramide
Dofetilide	Domperidone	Droperidol	Erythromycin
Halofantrine	Haloperidol	Ibutilide	Mesoridazine
Methadone	Pentamidine	Pimozide	Procainamide
Quinidine	Sotalol	Sparfloxacin	Thioridazine

Source: Arizona Center for Education and Research on Therapeutics 2008[274]

Antiretrovirals
Many antiretroviral medications interact with methadone and buprenorphine, see Table A5.2 and Table A5.3.

Other agents
St John's wort (Hypericum) is also a CYP3A4 inducer.

CYP450 inhibitors

Antifungals
Azole agents including ketoconazole, fluconazole and itraconazole, are potent inhibitors of CYP3A4 and have increased the effects of both methadone and buprenorphine. Prophylactic dose reductions should be considered.

Antiretrovirals
Many antiretroviral medications interact with methadone and buprenorphine, see Table A6.2 and Table A6.3.

Macrolide antibiotics
Most macrolides (erythromycin, clarithromycin, dirithromycin, roxithromycin) inhibit CYP3A4. Only azithromycin does not inhibit CYP3A4.

Other agents
Grapefruit juice is also a significant inhibitor of cytochrome P450 enzymes.

Table A5.2 Interactions between antiretroviral agents and methadone

Antiretroviral agent	Effect on methadone	Methadone effect on antiretroviral agent	Comment
Nucleoside/Nucleotide reverse transcriptase inhibitors (NRTIs)			
Abacavir (ABC)	Methadone clearance increased by 22%	Concentrations slightly decreased (but not clinically significant)	Patients should be monitored for methadone withdrawal symptoms; dose increase unlikely, but may be required in a small number of patients
Didanosine (ddI)	None	Buffered ddI concentration decreased by 57% EC ddI unchanged	Buffered ddI dose increase may be considered or use EC ddI in preference
Emtricitabine (FTC)	None	None	No known interactions
Lamivudine (3TC)	None	None	No known interactions
Stavudine (d4T)	None	Methadone co-administration reduced stavudine AUC and Cmax by 23% and 44%, respectively	The clinical significance of a change in drug exposure of this magnitude is not certain
Tenofovir (TDF)	None	None	–
Zidovudine (AZT)	None	Concentration increased by 29–43%	Monitor for AZT adverse effects, in particular bone marrow suppression (especially anaemia).
Non-nucleoside reverse transcriptase inhibitors (NNRTIs)			
Efavirenz (EFV)	Decreased methadone Cmax (45%) and AUC (52%), withdrawal reported	None	Symptoms of withdrawal may develop after 3–7 days, requiring significant increases in the methadone dose
Etravirine (TMC-125)	No clinically significant effect	No clinically significant effect	Observe, but no dose adjustments are likely to be needed.
Nevirapine (NVP)	Decreased, withdrawal reported	None	Withdrawal symptoms frequent; generally occurring between 4 and 8 days after starting nevirapine; in case series of chronic methadone recipients initiating nevirapine, 50–100% increases in the daily methadone doses were required to treat opiate withdrawal
Protease inhibitors (PIs)			
Atazanavir (ATV)	None	None	--- (if RTV-boosted: see RTV#).
Darunavir (DRV)	None	None	--- (if RTV-boosted: see RTV#).
Fos-amprenavir (FPV)	Mildly decreases methadone levels	Decreased amprenavir levels	Monitor and titrate to methadone response as necessary. Possibility of reduced effectiveness of fos-amprenavir, or consider using an alternative agent.
Indinavir (IDV)	None	Non-clinically significant interaction	--- (if RTV-boosted: see RTV#).
Lopinavir/ritonavir (LPV/r)	Decreased significantly	None	Methadone withdrawal possible; monitor and titrate to methadone response as necessary
Nelfinavir (NFV)	Decreases methadone levels	Mildly decreased, but not clinically significant	Clinical withdrawal rarely reported; methadone dose modification unlikely
Ritonavir (RTV)	Decreases methadone concentrations even at boosting dosage	None	May require higher methadone dose, even if only booster doses of ritonavir used; observe closely for signs of methadone withdrawal
Saquinavir (SQV)	None	None	--- (if RTV-boosted: see RTV#).
Tipranavir (TPV)	None	None	--- (if RTV-boosted: see RTV#).
Integrase Inhibitors			
Maraviroc (MRV)	No data - potentially safe	No data - potentially safe	
Raltegravir (RAL)	None expected	None expected	

– = no comment; --- = unknown; AUC =area under the curve, EC = enteric coated; RTV = ritonavir; RTV-boosted = ritonavir used in combination with other medication
Table adapted from the Integrated Management of Adolescent and Adult Illness manual on HIV care in injecting drug users,[284] the Liverpool HIV Pharmacology Group web site [2], the 2006 World Health Organization antiretroviral therapy guidelines,[285] and the Department of Health and Human Services Guidelines for the use of Antiretrovirals Agents in HIV-1-Infected Adults and Adolescents.[286]

2   http://www.hiv-druginteractions.org/

Table A5.3 Interactions between antiretroviral agents and buprenorphine

Antiretroviral agent	Effect on buprenorphine	Buprenorphine effect on antiretroviral agent	Comment
Nucleoside/Nucleotide reverse transcriptase inhibitors (NRTIs)			
Abacavir (ABC)	---	---	Potential interaction that may require close monitoring, alteration of drug dosage or timing of administration
Didanosine (ddI)	None	None	–
Emtricitabine (FTC)	None	None	–
Lamivudine (3TC)	None	None	–
Stavudine (d4T)	None	None	–
Tenofovir (TDF)	None	None	–
Zidovudine (AZT)	None	None	–
Non-nucleoside reverse transcriptase inhibitors (NNRTIs)			
Efavirenz (EFV)	Decreased buprenorphine concentration	None	Observe; may need buprenorphine dose increase
Etravirine (TMC-125)	No data	No data	Observe
Nevirapine (NVP)	No data	No data	Observe
Protease Inhibitors (PIs)			
Atazanavir (ATV)	Increased buprenorphine effects	None	Observe; buprenorphine dose reduction may be necessary
Darunavir (DRV)	No data	No data	Observe
Fos-Amprenavir (FPV/APV)	No data	No data	Observe
Indinavir (IDV)	Potential for increased buprenorphine effects	No data	Observe; buprenorphine dose reduction may be necessary
Lopinavir/ritonavir (LPV/r)	No data	No data	Observe
Nelfinavir (NFV)	No data	No data	Observe
Ritonavir (RTV)	Potential for increased buprenorphine effects	No data	Observe; buprenorphine dose reduction may be necessary
Saquinavir (SQV)	Potential for increased buprenorphine effects	No data	Observe; buprenorphine dose reduction may be necessary
Tipranavir (TPV)	Potential for increased buprenorphine effects	No data	Observe; buprenorphine dose reduction may be necessary
Integrase Inhibitors			
Maraviroc (MRV)	No data – potentially safe	No data – potentially safe	
Raltegravir (RAL)	None expected	None expected	

– = no comment; --- = unknown; EC = enteric coated
Table adapted from the Integrated Management of Adolescent and Adult Illness manual on HIV care in injecting drug users,[284] the Liverpool HIV Pharmacology Group web site[3], the 2006 World Health Organization antiretroviral therapy guidelines,[285] and the Department of Health and Human Services Guidelines for the use of Antiretrovirals Agents in HIV-1-Infected Adults and Adolescents.[286]

---

3 http://www.hiv-druginteractions.org/

Annex 6 Alternatives for the treatment of opioid dependence not included in the current guidelines

A6.1 Heroin maintenance

> The limited evidence is inadequate to support any recommendations on heroin maintenance.

A Cochrane review of heroin prescription identified five RCTs comparing heroin with methadone[287]. It was not possible to draw definitive conclusions about the overall effectiveness of heroin prescription because the experimental studies available were not compatible. Heroin use in clinical practice is still a matter of research in most countries. Results favouring heroin treatment over methadone come from studies conducted in patients who have failed previous methadone treatments.

A6.2 Slow or sustained-release oral morphine

> The limited evidence is inadequate to support any recommendations on slow or sustained-release oral morphine.

Recent formulations of morphine can be used in once-daily doses for the treatment of chronic pain[288, 289, 290] and there have been a number of studies of these formulations in opioid dependence[210, 291, 292, 293]. The results of these trials are promising, demonstrating a long duration of action of morphine and comparable levels of self-reported heroin use to methadone treatment. The use of morphine in the treatment of addiction is complicated by difficulties in assessing heroin use and supervising doses.

A6.3 Levo-alpha-acetylmethadol

> Although still registered in the United States, levo-alpha-acetylmethadol (LAAM) has been withdrawn from the market by the manufacturer, due to the risk of life-threatening cardiac arrhythmias.

Levo-alpha-acetylmethadol (LAAM) is a long-acting opioid agonist approved for use as a maintenance treatment for opioid dependence. For persons in whom methadone and buprenorphine are not effective, LAAM offers an alternative effective medication. In a Cochrane review and recent RCT, LAAM was found to be better at suppressing heroin use than methadone[294, 295] but its use is, at present, limited by its effect of QT prolongation[296]. The active metabolite – nor-acetylmethadol – does not have the same effect on QT prolongation[131, 297], and may be a promising treatment alternative.

A6.4 Buprenorphine-naloxone combination

> The limited evidence is inadequate to support any recommendations on a buprenorphine–naloxone combination. However, the combination is likely to have similar efficacy to buprenorphine alone.

As with methadone, intravenous abuse of buprenorphine has been reported in many countries[119, 128, 298, 299, 300, 301, 302, 303]. Buprenorphine–naloxone comprises the partial agonist buprenorphine in combination with the opioid antagonist naloxone in a 4:1 ratio. It is hoped that by the addition of naloxone, the resulting product will be less subject to abuse by injection than buprenorphine alone. When the combination is taken sublingually, absorption of naloxone is minimal and the opioid agonist effects of buprenorphine should predominate. However, when buprenorphine–naloxone tablets are injected, naloxone will induce withdrawal in people dependent on opioids other than buprenorphine[269, 271, 304].

Efficacy of buprenorphine/naloxone in maintenance therapy for opioid dependence is described in three RCTs in comparing the combination with placebo[305] and clonidine[226], and comparing stepped combination-based treatment with methadone treatment alone[306]. Three trials investigating the efficacy of the combination with different counselling or medication-dispensing regimens have been published[307, 308, 309].

A6.5 Slow-release naltrexone implants and injections

> The limited evidence is inadequate to support any recommendations on slow-release naltrexone implants and injections.

Injectable, slow-release naltrexone formulations provide clinically significant opioid blockade for 3-6 weeks (depending on the dose) in early clinical research[310, 311, 312, 313, 314].

A number of naltrexone implants have been developed that can be inserted subcutaneously using local anaesthesia, either post withdrawal or as part of an antagonist withdrawal treatment. Subsequent implants are inserted at 1–3 months intervals. There are no RCTs to assess the effectiveness of naltrexone implants, although there are some promising reports[315, 316, 317, 318]. Local implant site allergies and infections have been described with implantable formulations.

Annex 7 Methadone and buprenorphine and international drug control conventions

The Single Convention on Narcotic Drugs, 1961 (as amended by the 1972 Protocol) and the Convention on Psychotropic Substances, 1971 contain specific control provisions for some psychoactive substances[321, 322]. Pursuant to these conventions, the Commission on Narcotic Drugs (CND) has the authority to decide, upon a recommendation from the World Health Organization, whether a substance should be scheduled as a narcotic drug or a psychotropic substance.

Methadone is currently scheduled as a "narcotic drug", falling under the Single Convention on Narcotic Drugs and buprenorphine as a "psychotropic substance", falling under the Convention on Psychotropic Substances.

The International Narcotics Control Board (INCB) is charged with monitoring the compliance by Governments with the above international treaties, ensuring on the one hand that controlled substances are available for medical and scientific use and on the other hand that diversion from licit sources to illicit traffic does not occur[321].

A7.1 Single Convention on Narcotic Drugs 1961

The Single Convention on Narcotic Drugs is the principal international treaty regulating the control of opioids. It seeks to limit exclusively to medical and scientific purposes the production, manufacture, export, import, distribution of, trade in, use and possession of narcotic drugs. Heroin, opium, morphine, oxycodone, methadone, and most other potent pharmaceutical opioids (with the exception of buprenorphine) are listed as narcotic drugs under the 1961 Single Convention.

To comply with the convention with regard to methadone, countries must:
- estimate the annual medical and scientific requirements for methadone and submit their estimates to the INCB for confirmation
- limit the total quantities of methadone manufactured and imported to the relevant estimates, taking into account the quantity exported
- ensure that methadone remains in the hands of licenced parties from the point of manufacture or importation to dispensing
- provide that methadone is dispensed against a medical prescription
- report to INCB on the amount of methadone imported, exported, manufactured and consumed and of stocks held
- maintain a system of inspection of manufacturers, exporters, importers, and wholesale and retail distributors of narcotic drugs and of medical and scientific institutions that use such substances; premises, stocks and records should be inspected
- in addition, a country has a responsibility to ensure that diversion and abuse of methadone is prevented.

National estimates of medical need for opioids

Every year, national drug regulatory authorities must prepare estimates of the requirements for methadone of their country during the following year. The estimates must be submitted to the INCB six months in advance of the period for which they apply, but supplementary estimates may be submitted at any time. INCB publishes changes in the estimates received from governments on a monthly basis, as a guide for exporting countries. The responsibility for determining the amounts of opioids necessary to meet the medical and scientific requirements in a country rests entirely with the national governments, but the INCB must be informed of the method used. The INCB establishes estimates of annual requirements for narcotic drugs for countries which fail to do so. In case an estimate is established by INCB, the competent authorities of the country concerned are informed by the Board and requested to review the established estimates.

Obtaining a supply of methadone

After a country has received confirmation of its estimate from the INCB, it may commence manufacture or import procedures. In both cases, it is vital that the supply is reliable as interruptions to the supply of methadone are distressing for patients and place them at high risk of relapse to illicit opioid use.

Domestic manufacture

Some, or all of the methadone needed may be manufactured by enterprises in the country itself, under the regulation of the government. Regulation of manufacture of opioids includes licensing, requirements for record keeping and reporting, secure storage, and quality control.

The import/export system

A specific sequence of steps is stipulated in the convention for the import and export of narcotic drugs, although additional requirements may vary from country to country. Importation and exportation of methadone can only take place with the approval of the national drug regulatory authorities, and within the limits of the total of the estimates for the importing country. A copy of the export authorization must accompany each shipment.

The import and export authorization shall state:
- the name of the drug
- the international non-proprietary name (INN) of the drug, if any
- the quantity of the drug to be imported or exported
- the name and address of the importer and exporter
- the period of validity of the authorization.

The export authorization shall also state the number and date of the import authorization and the authority by whom it has been issued.

The steps involved in the import/export process

The import/export process is outlined below in Figure A7.1. Many countries also have an authorization/certification procedure to prevent marketing of pharmaceutical products that are falsely labelled, counterfeit or substandard.

1. The entity wishing to import a substance controlled under the Single Convention applies to its regulatory authority for an import authorization.
2. The regulatory authority considers whether the company is properly licensed and whether the drug and amount are within the national estimate; if approved, an original import authorization and the appropriate number of copies are issued. One copy should be sent to the competent authorities of the exporting country. The original and one copy should be sent to the importer who will send the original to the exporter and will keep one copy for the Customs declaration. One copy should be sent to the Customs authorities of the importing country and an additional copy should be kept in the records of the importing country's competent authority.
3. The importer sends the original of the import authorization to the company responsible for the export of the substance.
4. The exporter applies to its drug regulatory authority for an export authorization.
5. The regulatory authority in the exporting country checks that an import authorization has been issued and that the exporter is properly licensed, and that the estimate of the importing country is sufficient; if the application is approved, an export authorization is issued.
6. The regulatory authority in the exporting country sends a copy of the export authorization to the regulatory authority in the importing country. Two copies should be provided to the exporter, one of which must accompany the consignment. One copy should be sent to the Customs authorities of the exporting country and an additional copy should be kept in the records of the exporting country's competent authority.
7. The exporter ships the drugs to the importer, along with the copy of the

export authorization.
8. The shipment must pass a customs inspection.
9. The importer sends the export authorization to its regulatory authority. The regulatory authority of the importing country shall return the accompanying export authorization to the regulatory authority of the exporting country with an endorsement certifying the amount actually imported.

Figure A7.1 Steps in opioid importation

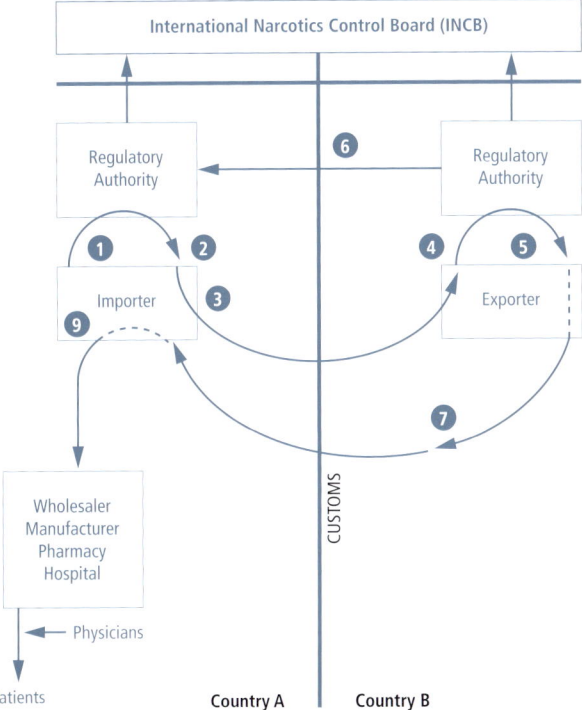

Adapted from WHO 1996[323]

The reporting system

National drug regulatory authorities must report to the INCB all imports and exports of methadone every quarter. They are also required to make an annual inventory and report the total amount of opioids manufactured, consumed and held in stock. The annual inventory does not include drugs stored in pharmacies, which for official purposes are considered to have been consumed.

Regulation of health-care workers

The convention recognizes that individual governments must decide the level of regulation of the individuals directly involved in dispensing opioids – pharmacists, physicians and nurses. However, it expresses several principles that should be observed:
- individuals must be authorized to dispense opioids by their professional licence to practice, or be specially licensed to do so
- movement of opioids may occur only between duly authorized parties
- a medical prescription is required before opioids may be dispensed to a patient.

Drug abuse versus patient need

The convention recognizes that governments have the right to impose further restrictions if they consider it necessary, to prevent diversion and misuse of opioids. However, this right must be continually balanced against the responsibility to ensure opioid availability for medical purposes.

In deciding the appropriate level of regulation, governments should bear in mind the dual aims of the convention. The INCB has observed that, in some countries, fear of drug abuse has resulted in laws and regulations, or interpretations of laws and regulations, which make it unnecessarily difficult to obtain opioids for medical use.

"…prevention of availability of many opiates for licit use does not necessarily guarantee the prevention of the abuse of illicitly procured opiates. Thus, an overly restrictive approach to the licit availability of opiates may, in the end, merely result in depriving a majority of the population of access to opiate medications for licit purposes"[324].

A7.2 Convention on Psychotropic Substances, 1971

This convention establishes an international control system for psychotropic substances that balances their abuse potential and therapeutic value. Buprenorphine is listed as a psychotropic substance and is currently included in Schedule III of the convention.

To comply with the convention with regard to buprenorphine, countries must:
- ensure that buprenorphine remains in the hands of licensed parties from the point of manufacture or importation to dispensing;
- provide that buprenorphine is dispensed only with a medical prescription;
- prohibit the advertisement of buprenorphine to the general public;
- request that all operators manufacturing, trading or distributing buprenorphine keep records on each acquisition and disposal for at least two years;
- report to INCB on the amount of buprenorphine imported, exported and manufactured on an annual basis;
- maintain a system to inspect manufacturers, exporters, importers, and wholesale and retail distributors of psychotropic substances and of medical and scientific institutions that use such substances; premises, stocks and records should be inspected;
- ensure diversion and abuse of buprenorphine is prevented.

Domestic manufacture

Some or all of the buprenorphine needed by a country may be manufactured by domestic enterprises, under the regulation of the government. Regulation of manufacture of psychotropic substances includes licensing, requirements for record keeping and reporting. Provisions relating to manufacture of pharmaceutical products in general, such as secure storage, and quality control, also apply.

Regulation of health-care workers

The convention recognizes that individual governments must decide the level of regulation of the individuals directly involved in dispensing psychotropic substances (i.e. pharmacists, physicians and nurses). However, it expresses several principles that should be observed:
- individuals must be adequately qualified, and authorized to dispense psychotropic substances by their professional licence to practice, or be specially licensed to do so
- movement may occur only between duly authorized parties
- a medical prescription is required before psychotropic substances may be dispensed to a patient, except when individuals may lawfully obtain, use, dispense or administer such substances in the duly authorized exercise of therapeutic or scientific functions

- prescriptions need to be issued in accordance with sound medical practice and subject to regulation to protect public health and welfare, particularly the number of times such prescriptions may be refilled and the duration of their validity.

Drug abuse versus patient need

The convention recognizes that governments have the right to impose further restrictions if they consider such restrictions necessary to prevent diversion and misuse of psychotropic substances. However, this right must be continually balanced against the responsibility to ensure the availability of psychotropic substances for medical purposes.

Obtaining a supply of buprenorphine

Reliable supply of buprenorphine is vital because interruptions to the supply are distressing for patients and place them at high risk of relapse to illicit opioid use. Although not required by the convention, most exporting countries will adhere to the additional voluntary control measures recommended by ECOSOC (see below). In practice, all importing countries should remember that they might encounter difficulties obtaining buprenorphine if they do not have an assessment (a simplified estimate of the annual requirements for a psychotropic substance, see below) covering the amount to be imported and an import authorization or 'no objection' certificate for each separate import.

Assessment of medical needs for buprenorphine in accordance with ECOSOC resolution 1993/38

National drug regulatory authorities should prepare an assessment of the annual requirements for buprenorphine of their country. INCB recommends that this assessment should be revised at least every three years. The assessment or its revision can be submitted at any time. The responsibility for determining the amounts of buprenorphine necessary to meet the medical and scientific need in a country rests entirely with the national governments. INCB publishes changes in the assessments received from governments on a monthly basis, as a guide to exporting countries.

The import–export system

A specific sequence of steps is specified in the convention for the import and export of psychotropic substances. Additional requirements have been recommended by ECOSOC, and they are adhered to by most governments.

1. Mandatory controls foreseen by the convention

The convention foresees mandatory import–export authorizations only for substances included in Schedules I and II.

When exporting Schedule III substances, such as buprenorphine, exporters have to submit two copies of an export declaration to the competent authorities of the exporting country, and the third copy of the export declaration has to accompany the consignment. The government of the exporting country must forward the export declaration to the competent authorities of the importing country as soon as possible, but not later than 90 days after the date of the dispatch. Countries may require the importer to transmit the copy accompanying the consignment, duly endorsed stating the quantities received and the date of receipt, to the competent authorities of the importing country.

The export declaration must include:
- the international non-proprietary name (INN) of the substance, or failing such a name, the designation of the substance in the Schedule
- the quantity and pharmaceutical form in which the substance is exported, and, if in the form of a preparation, the name of the preparation
- the name and address of the importer
- the name and address of the exporter
- the date of the dispatch.

2. Voluntary controls foreseen by ECOSOC resolutions

In accordance with ECOSOC resolution 1996/30, most governments have extended the import–export authorization system to Schedule III and IV substances, including buprenorphine. An import can only take place with the approval of the national drug regulatory authorities of the importing country and should remain within the assessment for buprenorphine established by the importing country. Approved export authorizations must accompany each consignment.

The import authorization must include:
- the authorization number
- the date it was issued
- the authority by whom it has been issued
- the international non-proprietary name (INN) of the substance(s), or failing such a name, the designation of the substance(s) in the Schedule
- the pharmaceutical form and quantity of the substance(s), and, if in the form of a preparation, the name of the preparation
- the name and address of the importer
- the name and address of the exporter
- the period of validity of the authorization.

The steps involved in the import–export process, in accordance with the recommendations of the ECOSOC resolutions
- The entity wishing to import buprenorphine applies to its regulatory authority for an import authorization.
- The regulatory authority considers whether the entity is properly licensed and whether the substance and amount are within the assessment; if approved, an original import authorization or 'no objection' certificate and the appropriate number of copies are issued. (One copy should be sent to the competent authorities of the exporting country. The original and one copy should go to the importer who will send the original to the exporter and will keep one copy for the Customs declaration. One copy should go to the Customs authorities of the importing country and an additional copy should be kept in the records of the importing country's competent authority.)
- The importer sends the original of the import authorization or certificate to the company responsible for the export of the substance.
- The exporter applies to its drug regulatory authority for an export authorization.
- The regulatory authority of the exporting country checks that an import authorization has been issued and that the exporter is properly licensed, and that the assessment of the importing country is sufficient; if the application is approved, an export authorization is issued.
- The regulatory authority of the exporting country sends a copy of the export authorization to the regulatory authority of the importing country. Two copies should go to the exporter, one of which must accompany the consignment. One copy should go to the Customs authorities of the exporting country and an additional copy should be kept in the records of the exporting country's competent authority.
- The exporter ships the drugs to the importer, along with the copy of the export authorization.
- The consignment must pass a customs inspection.
- The importer sends the export authorization to its regulatory authority. After receiving the consignment, the importing authority shall return the accompanying export authorization to the regulatory authority of the exporting country with an endorsement certifying the amount actually imported.

A7.3 Guidelines for regulation of health professionals

It is understood that regulatory requirements for physicians, nurses and pharmacists to dispense opioids to patients will differ from country to country. However, the following are general criteria that can be used to develop a practical system.

1. Legal authority. Physicians, nurses and pharmacists should be legally empowered to prescribe, dispense and administer opioids to patients in accordance with local needs.
2. Accountability. They must dispense opioids for medical purposes only and must be held responsible in law if they dispense them for non-medical purposes.
3. Appropriate records must be kept. If physicians are required to keep records other than those associated with good medical practice, the extra work incurred should be practicable and should not impede medical activities. Hospitals and pharmacists must be legally responsible for safe storage and the recording of opioids received and dispensed. Records of each individual acquisition and disposal of opioids must be preserved for a period of not less than two years.
4. Reasonable record keeping and accountability provisions should not discourage health-care workers from prescribing or stocking adequate supplies of opioids.
5. Prescriptions. Legal requirements for prescriptions vary by jurisdiction; however, in general a prescription for opioid agonist maintenance therapy should specify the following:
    - name, address and telephone number of the prescribing doctor
    - name of the pharmacy
    - name and address of the patient
    - date of the prescription
    - preparation to be dispensed (i.e. methadone or buprenorphine)
    - dose to be dispensed in milligrams (words and numbers)
    - frequency of dispensing (daily, twice daily, alternate daily, three times a week)
    - start and end dates of the prescription
    - whether doses are to be supervised or taken away.
6. Patient access. Opioids should be available in locations that will be accessible to as many opioid-dependent patients as possible.
7. Medical decisions. Decisions concerning the type of drug to be used, the amount of the prescription and the duration of therapy are best made by medical professionals on the basis of the individual needs of each patient.

Annex 8 Priorities for research

This annex describes weaknesses and gaps revealed by a review of the evidence to support treatment, conducted during the preparation of these guidelines.

A8.1 Gaps in the evidence

Comparisons between opioid agonist maintenance, detoxification and opioid antagonist approaches

Few studies comparing naltrexone treatments with opioid agonist maintenance treatments were found. The only randomized trial to compare methadone or buprenorphine with naltrexone was conducted in intravenous buprenorphine users[142]. There were no studies comparing long-acting naltrexone formulations to opioid agonist treatment approaches.

No studies assessed the potential benefit to populations of having more than one treatment available (e.g. buprenorphine and methadone, or opioid antagonists and opioid agonists).

No randomized trials were conducted in specific populations (e.g. young people, people with short histories of dependence, people who do not inject and pregnant women) to compare approaches based on opioid detoxification with approaches based on opioid agonist maintenance treatment. Although evidence strongly favours opioid agonist approaches, opioid detoxification remains the most requested treatment in many settings.

Impact of treatment on HIV transmission

Well-conducted observational studies to evaluate the impact of pharmacological treatment on HIV transmission would be useful, because most randomized trials did not collect data on HIV risk practices and HIV transmission. In particular, more data on the impact of buprenorphine treatment on HIV transmission is needed, because this treatment is unsupervised in many settings.

Optimal doses

Although there are sufficient studies on the optimal doses of methadone to make recommendations, the same is not true for buprenorphine. Research is also needed on the optimal doses of methadone and buprenorphine in non-injecting drug users (e.g. opium smokers).

Supervised dosing in agonist maintenance treatment

For both methadone and buprenorphine, surprisingly little research has been conducted on the impact of dosing supervision on treatment outcome. This is a particularly important question given the widespread use of unsupervised buprenorphine treatment in several countries.

Antagonist treatment in different settings

There is a discrepancy between the modest benefits of oral naltrexone treatment in developed countries and reports from clinicians of the usefulness of naltrexone in developing countries. Further research on opioid antagonists in developing countries is needed.

Prescription opioid dependence

In many countries, the number of people with prescription opioid dependence now exceeds the number of people with illicit opioid dependence. More research is required on the use of opioid detoxification and agonist maintenance in this population, including the required degree of supervision.

Adolescence

The relative lack of research in young people and people with brief histories of opioid dependence is concerning, because this population may have the greatest capacity for change. More research is needed on psychosocial assistance, including family-based approaches, and on the relative merits of opioid agonist treatment and withdrawal, and antagonist treatment.

Pregnancy and breastfeeding

More research is required to establish the safety of buprenorphine and naltrexone for pregnant and breastfeeding women.

Outcomes of planned cessation of agonist maintenance treatment

More research is needed on when opioid agonist treatment can be stopped without leading to high rates of relapse. Studies comparing methods of cessation of agonist maintenance treatment are also required.

Psychosocial support

More research is needed on various psychosocial approaches to treatment, particularly the more social approaches, such as employment and residential programmes.

A8.2 Methodological issues in research

Study size

Many studies are too small to adequately address the questions being asked. This may reflect the difficulties in funding clinical trials in this population, and the relatively small sizes of many treatment centres. Larger studies are required on most topics. In addition, many studies replicate earlier trials despite there remaining gaps in the evidence. Treatment networks at international levels may be needed to coordinate large trials to answer simple questions, a method that has been used in many fields of medicine in recent decades.

Study duration

The follow-up period of most studies is too short, given that opioid dependence is a chronic condition.

Study design

Most randomized trials considered in this review did not use intention-to-treat analyses, and many did not document allocation concealment. Although it is difficult to blind study participants in studies of psychoactive medication, greater consideration should be given to the use of blinding in outcome assessment and in the statistical analysis.

Outcome measures

Intention-to-treat analysis includes both "in treatment" and "out of treatment" patients. Most calculations assume that all people who drop out of treatment return to baseline levels of drug use. In reality, some people will start another form of treatment and other people will no longer require treatment. Although treatment retention is an important proxy measure in the absence of other relevant outcomes, continuous retention in treatment and treatment status at follow-up should be regarded as a measure of exposure to the intervention, rather than as a health outcome.

Studies should instead focus on drug use, related risk behaviours (e.g. injection, sexual activity that could lead to disease transmission) and health outcomes. Health outcomes should include measures of psychological health and well-being, function or dysfunction, quality of life, mortality and, where appropriate, specific health conditions (e.g. HIV, hepatitis C, sexually transmitted diseases).

Given that developments are taking place in pharmacogenetics research, consideration should be given to the storage of blood samples for such analysis from clinical trial participants, with their consent.

The impact of drug use beyond the individual (e.g. family, carers and society) should also be considered. Data for social cost estimates (e.g. criminal activity, health-care use, income and receipt of government benefits) are lacking for many settings. Cost-effectiveness and cost–benefit analyses are also possible if the cost of treatment is measured.

A8.3 Programmatic and systems research

Most research on treatments for opioid dependence has used the individual patient as the unit of analysis. There is significant variability in the conduct of treatment for opioid dependence worldwide. Greater emphasis on the treatment programme and the treatment system may improve the capacity of treatment systems to become more efficient and effective. Suggested research topics include the choice of treatment settings (e.g. primary care), dosing mechanisms and integration with other treatment systems (e.g. HIV treatment programmes).

From a public health perspective, the highest priority is to reduce the gap between the number of people with opioid dependence and the number with access to effective treatments.

Annex 9 Background papers prepared for technical expert meetings to inform guideline development

These papers are available from the web site of the WHO Department of Mental Health and Substance Use.[4]

A Systematic Review of Observational Studies on Treatment of Opioid Dependence

Anna Maria Bargagli, Marina Davoli, Silvia Minozzi,
Simona Vecchi, and Carlo A Perucci
Department of Epidemiology, ASL RM E, Rome, Italy

Costing Resource Needs for Opioid Dependence Treatment

Dan Chisolm, WHO

Economic Evaluation of Interventions for Illicit Opioid Dependence: A Review of Evidence

Chris Doran
National Drug & Alcohol Research Centre
University of New South Wales, Australia

Opium Abuse and Its Management: Global Scenario

Rajat Ray, S.Kattimani and H.K.Sharma
National Drug Dependence Treatment Centre
All India Institute of Medical Sciences
New Delhi, India

Psychosocially Assisted Pharmacotherapy for Opioid Dependence in Adolescents: A Review of the Existing Literature

Lisa A Marsch, Ph.D.
National Development and Research Institutes, Inc
United States

Psychosocial Interventions in Pharmacotherapy of Opioid Dependence: a Literature Review

Professor D Colin Drummond, MBChB, MD, FRCPsych
Professor of Addiction Psychiatry
Miss Katherine Perryman, BSc (Hons), MSc

---

4 http://www.who.int/substance_abuse/activities/third_meeting_tdg_opioid_dependence/en/index.html

Research Fellow
National Addiction Centre, UK

Review of the Literature on Pregnancy and Psychosocially Assisted Pharmacotherapy of Opioid Dependence (Including Withdrawal Management, Agonist and Antagonist Maintenance Therapy and Adjuvant Pharmacotherapy)

Univ. Prof. Dr Gabriele Fischer
Nina Kopf, cand.med.
Medical University of Vienna, Austria

Systematic Review of the Safety of Buprenorphine, Methadone and Naltrexone

Andy Gray
Department of Therapeutics and Medicines Management
Nelson R Mandela School of Medicine
University of KwaZulu-Natal
Durban, South Africa

The Ethical Use of Psychosocially Assisted Pharmacological Treatments for Opioid Dependence

Adrian Carter
Queensland Brain Institute
University of Queensland
Wayne Hall
School of Population Health
University of Queensland, Australia

The Role of Supervision of Dosing in Opioid Maintenance Treatment

James Bell, MD, FRACP, FAChAM
National Addiction Centre, London, United Kingdom

WHO Guidelines for Psychosocially Assisted Pharmacological Treatment of Persons Dependent on Opioids: Background Paper Prepared for the Ad-hoc Expert Meeting Geneva 1–4 November 2005

A Uchtenhagen, T Ladjevic, J Rehm
Research Institute for Public Health and Addiction
at Zurich University
Centre for Addiction and Mental Health
Toronto, Canada

Annex 10 Opioid withdrawal scales

Objective Opiate Withdrawal Scale (OOWS)

Observe the patient during a **5 minute observation period** then indicate a score for each of the opioid withdrawal signs listed below (items 1-13). Add the scores for each item to obtain the total score

Date

Time

1. **Yawning**
   0 = no yawns
   1 = ≥ 1 yawn

2. **Rhinorrhoea**
   0 = < 3 sniffs
   1 = ≥ 3 sniffs

3. **Piloerection** (observe arm)
   0 = absent
   1 = present

4. **Perspiration**
   0 = absent
   1 = present

5. **Lacrimation**
   0 = absent
   1 = present

6. **Tremor** (hands)
   0 = absent
   1 = present

7. **Mydriasis**
   0 = absent
   1 = ≥ 3 mm

8. **Hot and cold flushes**
   0 = absent
   1 = shivering / huddling for warmth

9. **Restlessness**
   0 = absent
   1 = frequent shifts of position

10. **Vomiting**
    0 = absent
    1 = present

11. **Muscle twitches**
    0 = absent
    1 = present

12. **Abdominal cramps**
    0 = absent
    1 = holding stomach

13. **Anxiety**
    0 = absent
    1 = mild - severe

    TOTAL SCORE

Source: Handelsman et al 1987[325]

Subjective Opiate Withdrawal Scale (SOWS)

In the column below in today's date and time, and in the column underneath, write in a number from 0-4 corresponding to how you feel about each symptom RIGHT NOW.
Scale: 0 = not at all 1 = a little 2 = moderately 3 = Quite a bit 4 = extremely

Date

Time

	Symptom	Score	Score	Score	Score	Score	Score
1	I feel anxious						
2	I feel like yawning						
3	I am perspiring						
4	My eyes are teary						
5	My nose is running						
6	I have goosebumps						
7	I am shaking						
8	I have hot flushes						
9	I have cold flushes						
10	My bones and muscles ache						
11	I feel restless						
12	I feel nauseous						
13	I feel like vomiting						
14	My muscles twitch						
15	I have stomach cramps						
16	I feel like using now						
	TOTAL						

Source: Handelsman et al 1987[325]

Clinical Opiate Withdrawal Scale (COWS)

For each item, circle the number that best describes the patient's signs or symptom. Rate on just the apparent relationship to opiate withdrawal. For example, if heart rate is increased because the patient was jogging just prior to assessment, the increase pulse rate would not add to the score.

Patient's Name:_____ Date and Time ____/____/____:_____
Reason for this assessment:_____

Resting Pulse Rate:_____beats/minute
Measured after patient is sitting or lying for one minute
0   pulse rate 80 or below
1   pulse rate 81-100
2   pulse rate 101-120
4   pulse rate greater than 120

Sweating: *over past ½ hour not accounted for by room temperature or patient activity.*
0   no report of chills or flushing
1   subjective report of chills or flushing
2   flushed or observable moistness on face
3   beads of sweat on brow or face
4   sweat streaming off face

Restlessness *Observation during assessment*
0   able to sit still
1   reports difficulty sitting still, but is able to do so
3   frequent shifting or extraneous movements of legs/arms
5   Unable to sit still for more than a few seconds

Pupil size
0   pupils pinned or normal size for room light
1   pupils possibly larger than normal for room light
2   pupils moderately dilated
5   pupils so dilated that only the rim of the iris is visible

Bone or Joint aches *If patient was having pain previously, only the additional component attributed to opiates withdrawal is scored*
0   not present
1   mild diffuse discomfort
2   patient reports severe diffuse aching of joints/ muscles
4   patient is rubbing joints or muscles and is unable to sit still because of discomfort

Runny nose or tearing *Not accounted for by cold symptoms or allergies*
0   not present
1   nasal stuffiness or unusually moist eyes
2   nose running or tearing
4   nose constantly running or tears streaming down cheeks

GI Upset: *over last ½ hour*
0   no GI symptoms
1   stomach cramps
2   nausea or loose stool
3   vomiting or diarrhea
5   Multiple episodes of diarrhea or vomiting

Tremor *observation of outstretched hands*
0   No tremor
1   tremor can be felt, but not observed
2   slight tremor observable
4   gross tremor or muscle twitching

Yawning *Observation during assessment*
0   no yawning
1   yawning once or twice during assessment
2   yawning three or more times during assessment
4   yawning several times/minute

Anxiety or Irritability
0   none
1   patient reports increasing irritability or anxiousness
2   patient obviously irritable anxious
4   patient so irritable or anxious that participation in the assessment is difficult

Gooseflesh skin
0   skin is smooth
3   piloerrection of skin can be felt or hairs standing up on arms
5   prominent piloerrection

Total Score _____
The total score is the sum of all 11 items

Initials of person
completing Assessment: _____

Score: 5-12 = mild; 13-24 = moderate; 25-36 = moderately severe; more than 36 = severe withdrawal
Source: Wesson and Ling 2003[326]

Modified Finnegan Scale

This scale is used for the measurement of neonatal abstinence syndrome due to neonatal opioid withdrawal.

Date and Time in Hours

System	Signs and Symptoms	Score								
Central Nervous System Disturbances	High-Pitched Cry	2								
	Continuous High-Pitched Cry	3								
	Sleeps<1 hour after feeding	3								
	Sleeps<2 hours after feeding	2								
	Sleeps>3 hours after feeding	1								
	Mild Tremors Disturbed	1								
	Mod-Severe Tremors Disturbed	2								
	Mild Tremors Undisturbed	3								
	Mod-Severe Tremors Undisturbed	4								
	Increased Muscle Tone	2								
	Excoriation (specify area)	1								
	Myoclonic Jerks	3								
	Generalised Convulsions	5								
Metabolic/Vasomotor/ Respiratory Disturbances	Fever (37.3°C-38.3°C)	1								
	Fever (38.4°C and higher)	2								
	Frequent Yawning (>3.4 times)	1								
	Nasal Stuffiness	1								
	Sneezing (>3-4 times)	1								
	Nasal Flaming	2								
	Respiratory Rate > 60/min	1								
	Respiratory Rate >60/min with retractions	2								
Gastrointestinal Disturbances	Excessive sucking	1								
	Poor Feeding	2								
	Regurgitation	2								
	Projectile Vomiting	3								
	Loose Stools	2								
	Watery Stools	3								
	Mas Score:41 Total Score									
	Scorer's Initials									

Neonatal Withdrawal Scoring Chart (Term infants)

Source: Finnegan 1980.[327]

Neonatal Abstinence Syndrome Scoring Chart

Guidelines for Neonatal Abstinence Syndrome (NAS) Scoring

Score 1 for each of the following (except 1).
1. **High pitched cry:** Score 2 if a cry is high-pitched at its peak, score 3 if a cry is high-pitched throughout.
2. **Sleep:** Consider total amount of time baby was asleep between feeds.
3. **Tremors:** This is a scale of increasing severity, and only one score should be made from the four categories. Undisturbed sleep means when the baby is asleep or at rest in a cot.
4. **Increased muscle tone:** Score if the baby has a generalised muscle tone greater than the upper limit of normal.
5. **Excoriation:** Score if skin excoriation occurs more than three to four times in 30 minutes.
6. **Nasal flaring:** Score if nasal flaring is present without other evidence of airways disease.
7. **Respiratory rate:** Score if respiratory rate of greater than 60 per minute is present without other evidence of airways disease.
8. **Excessive sucking:** Score if the baby sucks more than average.
9. **Poor feeding:** Score if the baby is very slow to feed or takes inadequate amounts.
10. **Regurgitation:** Score only if the baby regurgitates more frequently than usual in newborn infants.

Modifications for prematurity are mainly necessary in the sections on sleeping, e.g. a baby who needs three-hourly feeds can only sleep at most 2.5 hours between them. Scoring should be 1 if the baby sleeps less than two, 2 if sleeps less than one hour, and 3 if the baby does not sleep between feeds. Many premature babies require tube feeding. Babies should not be scored for poor feeding if tube feeding is customary for their period of gestation.

If the baby has three consecutive scores averaging more than eight (8), the child should be treated for NAS.

Annex 11 Summary of characteristics of selected psychoactive substances

Substance	Primary mechanism of action	Behavioural effects	Tolerance	Withdrawal	Effects of prolonged use
Ethanol	Increases activity of GABA-A receptors	Sedation Impaired memory Motor incoordination Anxiolysis	Metabolic tolerance occurs due to enzyme induction Behavioural tolerance develops through learning Tolerance also develops through changes to GABA-A receptor	Shaking, perspiration, weakness, agitation, headache, nausea, vomiting Seizures Delirium tremens	Altered brain function and morphology Cognitive impairments Decreased brain volume
Hypnotics and sedatives	Benzodiazepines: facilitate GABA's opening of GABA-A chloride channel Barbiturates: bind to a specific site on the GABA ionophore and increase chloride conductance	Sedation Anaesthesia Motor incoordination Cognitive impairments Memory impairment	Develops rapidly to most effects (except anticonvulsant) due to changes in GABA-A receptor	Anxiety, arousal, restlessness, insomnia, excitability, seizures	Memory impairment
Nicotine	Nicotinic cholinergic receptor agonist Increases sodium inflow through the channel, causing depolarization	Arousal, increased attention; concentration and memory; decreased anxiety, decreased appetite, stimulant-like effects	Tolerance develops through metabolic factors, as well as receptor changes	Irritability, hostility, anxiety, dysphoria, depressed mood, decreased heart rate, increased appetite	Health effects due to smoking are well-documented Difficult to dissociate effects of nicotine from other components of tobacco
Opioids	Mu and delta opioid receptor agonists	Euphoria, analgesia, sedation, respiratory depression	Short-term and long-term receptor desensitization Adaptations in intracellular signalling mechanisms	Watering eyes, runny nose, yawning, sweating, restlessness, chills, cramps, muscle aches	Long-term changes in opioid receptors and peptides Adaptations in reward, learning, stress responses
Cannabinoids	CB1 receptor agonists	Relaxation, increased sensory awareness, decreased short-term memory, motor incoordination, analgesia, antiemetic and antiepileptic effects, increased appetite	Develops rapidly to most effects	Rare, perhaps due to long half-life of cannabinoids	Cognitive impairments, risk of relapse and exacerbation of mental illness
Cocaine	Monoamine (dopamine, norepinephrine, serotonin) transporter blocker (increases monoamines in synaptic cleft)	Increased alertness, energy, motor activity, feelings of competence; euphoria, anxiety, restlessness, paranoia	Perhaps short-term acute tolerance	Not much, except "post-high down"	Cognitive deficits, Abnormalities on PET with orbitofrontal cortex Impaired motor function Decreased reaction times EEG abnormalities Cerebral ischaemia, infarcts, haemorrhages
Amphetamines	Increased release of dopamine from nerve terminals via dopamine transporter Not dependent upon action potentials Inhibits monoamine oxidase (MAO)	Increased alertness, arousal, energy, motor activity, speech, self-confidence, concentration, feelings of well-being; decreased hunger, increased heart rate, increased respiration, euphoria	Develops rapidly to behavioural and physiological effects	Fatigue, increased appetite, irritability, emotional depression, anxiety	Sleep disturbances, anxiety, decreased appetite, increased blood pressure; decreased brain dopamine, precursors, metabolites and receptors
Ecstasy	Blocks serotonin reuptake	Increased self-confidence, empathy, understanding, sensations of intimacy, increased communication, euphoria, increased energy	May develop in some individuals	Nausea, muscle stiffness, headache, loss of appetite, blurred vision, dry mouth, insomnia, depression, anxiety, fatigue, difficulty concentrating	Neurotoxic to brain serotonin systems, leads to behavioural and physiological consequences
Volatile solvents	Most likely GABA-A receptor mediated	Dizziness, disorientation, euphoria, light-headedness, increased mood, hallucinations, delusions, incoordination, visual disturbances, anxiolysis, sedation	Some tolerance develops (difficult to estimate)	Increased susceptibility to seizures	Changes in dopamine receptor binding and function Decreased cognitive function Psychiatric and neurological sequelae
Hallucinogens	Varies: LSD: serotonin autoreceptor agonist PCP: NMDA glutamate receptor antagonist Atropinics: muscarinic cholingergic receptor antagonists	Increased heart rate, blood pressure, body temperature; decreased appetite, nausea, vomiting, motor incoordination, papillary dilatation, hallucinations	Tolerance develops rapidly to physical and psychological effects	No evidence	Acute or chronic psychotic episodes, flashbacks or re-experiencing of drug effects long after drug use

Source: WHO 2004[9]

Annex 12 Prescribing guidelines

Specific cautions regarding the use of methadone and buprenorphine

Intoxicated or sedated patients

Methadone and buprenorphine should not be given to patients showing signs of intoxication or sedation, due to the risk of sedative overdose. The risks of methadone and buprenorphine use in opioid-dependent patients who are frequently intoxicated with sedatives such as alcohol and benzodiazepines, needs to be balanced against the benefits of treatment.

Severe hepatic/renal dysfunctions

The metabolism and elimination of methadone and buprenorphine may be affected by either hepatic or renal dysfunction in which case the dose or dosing frequency should be adjusted accordingly.

Respiratory insufficiency

In patients with respiratory insufficiency, methadone and buprenorphine may reduce the respiratory drive.

Psychosis

In patients with active psychosis the risks and benefits of methadone and buprenorphine need to be carefully considered.

Methadone maintenance treatment

Induction

The initial daily dose of methadone should depend on the level of neuroadaptation to opioids. It should generally not be more than 20 mg, except in cases of higher tolerance to opioids, and even then should not be more than 30 mg. For people with low or uncertain levels of tolerance to opioids, the initial daily dose should be 10–15 mg. Caution should be exercised with initial methadone doses more than 20 mg daily. Observing patients 2–3 hours after their dose enables the best assessment of the degree of tolerance to opioids. If patients have significant opioid withdrawal symptoms 2–3 hours after their dose of methadone, then they should be given an additional 5–10 mg methadone and a corresponding increase in their next daily dose. If patients are sedated after their dose of methadone, then the next daily dose should be reduced (and the patient monitored until they are no longer sedated, or treated for overdose, if necessary).

Patients should be observed each day prior to dosing. Patients who are sedated or intoxicated should not be given further doses methadone until the sedation has abated.

Precautions for commencing methadone include: high-risk polydrug use, mental illness, low levels of neuroadaptation to opioids (i.e. recent incarceration), and significant concomitant medical problems.

Stabilization

Once patients are taking opioid agonist maintenance treatment without intoxication or significant withdrawal symptoms, the aim is to titrate the methadone dose to its most effective level. The daily dose of methadone should then be increased by 5–10 mg every few days, as needed, to reduce cravings for opioids, and illicit opioid use. The dose should not be increased by more than 20 mg per week.

Patients should be reviewed prior to each dose increase.

The average effective dose of methadone is 60–120 mg.

Switching from buprenorphine to methadone

Commence methadone 24 hours after the last dose of buprenorphine. From buprenorphine doses of 8 mg daily and above, commence with 30 mg methadone daily. From buprenorphine doses of 4-8 mg daily, commence with 20-30 mg methadone daily. With buprenorphine doses below 4 mg daily, commence with less than 20 mg methadone daily.

Missed methadone doses

If one of two doses are missed the patient can be maintained on the same methadone dose.

If three doses are missed the next methadone dose should be reduced by 25% to adjust for the possible reduction in tolerance. If it is well tolerated, doses can return to previous dose levels. If four doses are missed the next dose should be reduced by 50% to adjust for the potential reduction in tolerance. If the dose is well tolerated doses can be increased over several days to previous levels. If more than four doses are missed, patients should resume induction from baseline.

Frequency of doses

Methadone can be administered daily for most patients. In approximately 30% of patients, methadone does not produce effects that are evenly sustained over 24 hours. This can also occur in pregnancy and when methadone is used in combination with medications that increase its metabolism. In such cases methadone can be administered twice a day, dividing the dose in two. When it is too difficult to pick up the medication twice a day, or when take-home doses are not suitable, then buprenorphine should be considered. Increasing the dose of methadone will increase the duration of action to some extent, but the main determinant is the rate of metabolism of methadone.

Reducing dosage and stopping treatment.

The decision to discontinue therapy with methadone should be made as part of a comprehensive treatment plan. Evidence suggests that it is associated with a risk of relapse to illicit opioid use and patients should be informed of these risks. Research is lacking on factors predicting successful withdrawal from agonist maintenance, however these may include a brief drug-use history prior to opioid agonist maintenance, no previous treatments prior to opioid agonist treatment, current employment, stable accommodation, cessation of illicit opioid use, cessation of other drug use (including cannabis), and a positive change of social and physical environment since starting treatment.

The daily dose can be generally reduced by up to 2.5 to 5 mg per week without severe opioid withdrawal symptoms. Patients should be reviewed frequently during dose reductions and adjustments to the dose made in accordance with clinical need.

Methadone for opioid detoxification

Commence with 10-20 mg methadone daily, according to the severity of dependence and degree of tolerance to opioids. Reduce the daily methadone dose by 1–2 mg per day. Patients will continue to experience mild opioid withdrawal symptoms in the week after methadone is ceased.

Buprenorphine maintenance treatment

Induction

An adequate maintenance dose, titrated to clinical effectiveness, should be achieved as rapidly as possible to prevent undue opioid withdrawal symptoms due to inadequate dosage.

Prior to induction, consideration should be given to the nature of opioids being used (i.e. long or short-acting), the time since last opioid use, and the degree or level of opioid dependence (i.e. opioid tolerance).

Patients taking street heroin (or other short-acting opioids). When treatment starts, the dose of buprenorphine should be taken at least six hours after the patient last used opioids, or when the early signs of withdrawal appear. The recommended starting dose is 4 mg buprenorphine on day 1, with a possible additional 4 mg depending on the individual patient's requirement.

Patients on methadone. Before starting treatment with buprenorphine, the maintenance dose of methadone should be reduced to 30 mg/day. The first dose of buprenorphine should be taken at least 24 hours after the patient last used methadone. The initial 4 mg buprenorphine induction dose should ideally be administered when withdrawal signs are evident.

Precautions for commencing buprenorphine include: high-risk polydrug use, mental illness, low levels of neuroadaptation to opioids (i.e. recent incarceration), and significant concomitant medical problems.

Stabilization

The dose of buprenorphine should be increased progressively according to the clinical effect in the individual patient. It is recommended to use 8–24 mg daily, the daily dose should not exceed 32 mg. The dosage is adjusted according to reassessments of the clinical and psychological status of the patient.

Less than daily dosing with buprenorphine

After a satisfactory period of stabilization has been achieved the frequency of dosing may be decreased to dosing every other day at twice the individually titrated daily dose. For example, a patient stabilized to receive a daily dose of 8 mg may be given 16 mg on alternate days, with no medication on the intervening days. However, the dose given on any one day should not exceed 32 mg.

In some patients, after a satisfactory period of stabilization has been achieved, the frequency of dosing may be decreased to three times a week (for example on Monday, Wednesday and Friday). The dose on Monday and Wednesday should be twice the individually titrated daily dose, and the dose on Friday should be three times the individually titrated daily dose, with no medication on the intervening days. However, the dose given on any one day should not exceed 32 mg.

Transfer to methadone

Commence methadone 24 hours after the last dose of buprenorphine. From buprenorphine doses of 8 mg daily and above, commence with 30 mg methadone daily. From buprenorphine doses of 4–8 mg daily, commence with 20–30 mg methadone daily. With buprenorphine doses below 4 mg daily, commence with less than 20mg methadone daily.

Reducing dosage and stopping treatment

The decision to discontinue therapy with buprenorphine should be made as part of a comprehensive treatment plan. Studies suggest that it is associated with a risk of relapse to illicit opioid use and patients should be informed of these risks. Research is lacking on factors predicting successful withdrawal from opioid agonist maintenance; however, these factors may include a brief drug-use history before opioid agonist maintenance, no previous treatments before opioid agonist treatment, current employment, stable accommodation, cessation of illicit opioid use, cessation of other drug use (including cannabis), and a positive change of social and physical environment since starting treatment.

The daily dose of buprenorphine can generally be reduced by up to 4–8 mg per week without severe opioid withdrawal symptoms. Patients should be reviewed frequently during dose reductions and adjustments to the dose made in accordance with clinical need.

Buprenorphine for opioid detoxification

Different dose schedules have been used for detoxification from opioids using buprenorphine. One suggested schedule is:

- Day 1   6 mg
- Day 2   10 mg +/- 2 mg
- Day 3   10 mg +/- 2 mg
- Day 4   8 mg +/- 2 mg
- Day 5   4 mg.

Alpha 2 adrenergic agonists for opioid detoxification

Alpha adrenergic agonists can cause significant hypotension and bradycardia and should not be the treatment of choice for the management of opioid withdrawal in elderly patients and patients with coronary insufficiency, ischaemic heart disease, bradycardia, cerebrovascular disease, pregnancy and breastfeeding. It is recommended to monitor the pulse and blood pressure when using clonidine, and to withhold or reduce the dose if the patient experiences symptoms of reduced circulation (e.g. dizziness on standing) or if the pulse or the blood pressure become too low (e.g. pulse less than 50 bpm, blood pressure less than 90/60 mmHg).

Clonidine

In the management of opioid withdrawal, clonidine is generally administered in doses of up to 100–300 mcg, three or four times daily, up to a maximum of 10–17 mcg/kg/day, reducing after the first two days and finishing by day 4 or 5. In an inpatient or residential setting, the initial dose should be in the range of 1–2 mcg/kg, with subsequent doses adjusted accordingly.

In outpatient settings, where blood pressure is not being monitored, lower doses should be used, with maximum daily doses of 450–900 mcg, according to the patient's weight and severity of opioid withdrawal.

Lofexidine

Initially the dose is 0.4–0.6 mg twice daily, increasing as necessary and tolerated to a maximum of 2.4 mg daily, in 2–4 divided doses. Treatment should be for 7–10 days, followed by a gradual withdrawal of 2–4 days.

Guanfacine

Initially the dose should be 0.25 to 0.5 mg per day, increased as necessary and tolerated to 1-2 mg daily (in 1–4 divided doses) for 3–5 days then tapering over 2–3 days.

Other treatments for opioid withdrawal

Many different medications can be used in combination with alpha-2 agonists to manage specific symptoms of opioid withdrawal (e.g. benzodiazepines for anxiety and insomnia, anti-emetics for nausea and vomiting, and paracetamol and non-steroidal anti-inflammatory drugs [NSAIDs] for muscle aches). Detailed guidance on the use of these medications is beyond the scope of these guidelines.

Patients with diarrhoea, vomiting and excessive sweating can become significantly dehydrated and occasionally aggressive fluid replacement may be required.

Naltrexone treatment

Induction phase

Naltrexone commences after detoxification and after the patient has been free of opioids for 7 days (for short-acting opioids) or 10 days (for methadone). This should be verified at least by a negative urine drug screen and also by a negative naloxone challenge test, if in doubt. The standard maintenance dose is 50 mg orally per day. If patients experience gastrointestinal side effects, these may be helped by reducing the dose to 25 mg naltrexone for a few days.

Maintenance phase

If patients use heroin on a day that they have taken naltrexone, they can continue to take naltrexone the next day.

If a patient misses a day of naltrexone and takes heroin or other opioids, they should either recommence naltrexone at the earliest opportunity or wait 7 days and recommence as per normal induction. If they recommence naltrexone straight away they will experience a reduced withdrawal syndrome. To predict the severity of the withdrawal syndrome, patients can be given a naloxone challenge. Alpha-2 adrenergic agonists can be used to manage the withdrawal symptoms that occur.

If a patient misses more than one day of naltrexone and takes heroin or other opioids, they may experience severe opioid withdrawal upon naltrexone recommencement and patients should be advised to wait 7 days or alternatively to consider opioid agonist maintenance therapy.

There is no good evidence on the optimal duration of treatment. It is recommended that this be individually determined according to the specific clinical situation.

Naltrexone can be ceased without a withdrawal syndrome. Commencing opioid agonist maintenance therapy from naltrexone should proceed with great caution because the tolerance to opioids will be very low.

Annex 13 Glossary

Abstinence

Refraining from drug use. A person taking prescribed methadone but no illicit opioids would still be described as abstinent. The term "abstinence" should not be confused with the term "abstinence syndrome", which refers to withdrawal syndrome.

Agonist maintenance therapy, opioid

Treatment of drug dependence by prescribing a substitute drug to which the patient is cross-dependent and cross-tolerant. Examples of agonist maintenance therapies are methadone and buprenorphine to treat heroin dependence, and nicotine gum to replace tobacco smoking. The goals of agonist maintenance therapy are to eliminate or reduce use of a particular substance (especially if it is illegal), reduce the harm and health risks of a particular method of substance administration (e.g. risk of disease from needle-sharing) and reduce the social consequences of drug dependence. Agonist maintenance therapy can last from several months to more than 20 years, and is often accompanied by other treatment (e.g. psychosocial treatment). It is sometimes distinguished from tapering-off therapy. (See opioid withdrawal syndrome.)

Bloodborne diseases

Diseases such as HIV and hepatitis B and C, which are spread by blood-to-blood contact (e.g. needle sharing).

Convention on Psychotropic Substances, 1971

The Convention on Psychotropic Substances, 1971 is the second of the international drug control treaties, supplementing the Single Convention on Narcotic Drugs, 1961. It aims to control psychotropic substances, as defined under this convention, and to prevent their abuse. The Convention outlines a number of responsibilities for parties. The International Narcotics Control Board (INCB), which submits its reports to the Economic and Social Council (ECOSOC) through the Commission on Narcotics Drugs (CND) is responsible for monitoring the compliance by governments with the 1971 Convention, ensuring on the one hand that psychotropic substances are available for medical and scientific use, and on the other hand that diversion from licit sources to illicit traffic does not occur. Buprenorphine is listed in the Convention on Psychotropic Substances.

Dependence

As a general term, the state of needing or depending on something or someone for support or to function or survive. As applied to opioids, implies the need for repeated doses of a drug to feel good or to avoid feeling bad.

In 1964, a World Health Organization (WHO) Expert Committee introduced the term "dependence" to replace addiction and habituation. The term can generally be used with reference to dependence on any psychoactive drugs (e.g. drug dependence, chemical dependence, substance dependence), or with specific reference to a particular drug or class of drugs (e.g. opioid dependence). Although ICD-10 has a specific definition for dependence, described in terms applicable across drug classes, the symptoms of dependence will vary for each specific drug.

Dependence often refers to both the physical and psychological elements of drug dependence. More specifically, psychological or psychic dependence refers to the experience of impaired control over drug use (including cravings and compulsions to use drugs) while physiological or physical dependence refers to tolerance and withdrawal symptoms (see neuroadaptation). However, in biologically oriented discussion, dependence is often used to refer only to physical dependence.

Dependence or physical dependence is also used in a narrower sense in the psychopharmacological context, to refer solely to the development of withdrawal symptoms on cessation of drug use.

Detoxification

The process of an individual being withdrawn from the effects of a psychoactive substance. When referring to a clinical procedure, detoxification refers to a withdrawal process that is carried out in a safe and effective manner, minimizing the withdrawal symptoms. The facility where this takes place may be called a detoxification or "detox" centre.

Harm reduction

In the context of alcohol or other drugs, harm reduction (or harm minimization) describes policies or programmes that focus directly on reducing the harm resulting from the use of alcohol or drugs. The term is used particularly to refer to policies or programmes that aim to reduce the harm without necessarily changing the underlying drug use; examples include needle and syringe exchanges to counteract needle sharing among heroin users, and self-inflating airbags in automobiles to reduce injury in accidents, particularly as a result of drink–driving. Harm-reduction strategies cover a wider range of activities than simple reduction of supply and demand.

Harmful use of opioids

A pattern of psychoactive substance use that is causing damage to health (ICD-10, code F11.1). The damage may be physical (e.g. in the cases of hepatitis from the self-administration of injected psychoactive substances) or mental. Harmful use often, but not always, has adverse social consequences; social consequences alone, however, are not sufficient to justify a diagnosis of harmful use.

The term was introduced in ICD-10 and replaced "non-dependent use" as a diagnostic term.

Narcotic drug

Narcotic drugs are the substances included in Schedules I and II of the Single Convention on Narcotic Drugs, 1961, (see below), whether natural or synthetic. Methadone is a narcotic drug.

Neuroadaptation

The changes in neurones associated with both tolerance and the appearance of withdrawal syndrome. Individuals can exhibit neuroadaptation without showing the cognitive or behavioural manifestation of dependence. For example, surgical patients given opioid substances to relieve pain may sometimes experience withdrawal symptoms but may not recognize these symptoms or have any desire to continue taking drugs.

Opiate

One of a group of alkaloids derived from the opium poppy (*Papaver somniferum*), with the ability to induce analgesia, euphoria, and, in higher doses, stupor, coma, and respiratory depression. The term excludes synthetic opioids.

Opioid

The generic term applied to alkaloids from the opium poppy (*Papaver somniferum*), their synthetic analogues, and compounds synthesized in the body. All of these substances interact with the same specific receptors in the brain, have the capacity to relieve pain and produce a sense of well-being (euphoria). The opium alkaloids and their synthetic analogues also cause stupor, coma and respiratory depression in high doses.

Opium alkaloids and their semisynthetic derivatives include morphine, diacetylmorphine (diamorphine, heroin), hydromorphine, codeine and oxycodone. Synthetic opioids include levorphanol, propoxyphene, fentanyl, methadone, pethidine (meperidine) and the agonist–antagonist pentazocine. Endogenously occurring compounds with opioid actions include the endorphins and enkephalins.

The most commonly used opioids (such as morphine, heroin, hydromorphone, methadone and pethidine) bind preferentially to the μ-receptors; they produce analgesia, mood changes (e.g. euphoria, which may change to apathy or dysphoria), respiratory depression, drowsiness, psychomotor retardation, slurred speech and impaired concentration, memory and judgement.

Physical consequences of opioid use (mostly resulting from intravenous administration) include hepatitis B, hepatitis C, HIV, septicaemia, endocarditis (inflammation of the inner layer of the heart), pneumonia and lung abscess, thrombophlebitis (blood clots causing vein inflammation) and rhabdomyolysis (breakdown of muscle fibres). Psychological and social impairment is common, reflecting the illicit nature of non-medical opioid use.

Opioid, endogenous

Any of the naturally occurring brain neuropeptides, which include at least two major groups–the enkephalins and the endorphins. Both can interact with opiate-binding sites (receptors) and thus may modulate the perception of pain. Endorphins also appear to modulate mood and responses to stressful stimuli (see opioid).

Opioid intoxication

A condition that follows the administration of opioids, resulting in disturbances in the level of consciousness, cognition, perception, judgement, affect, behaviour or other psychophysiological functions and responses. These disturbances are related to the acute pharmacological effects of, and learned responses to, opioids. With time, these disturbances resolve, resulting in complete recovery, except where tissue damage or other complications have arisen.

Intoxication depends on the type and dose of opioid, and is influenced by factors such as an individual's level of tolerance. Individuals often take drugs in the quantity required to achieve a desired degree of intoxication. Behaviour resulting from a given level of intoxication is strongly influenced by cultural and personal expectations about the effects of the drug.

Acute intoxication is the ICD-10 term for intoxication of clinical significance (F11.0). Complications may include trauma, inhalation of vomitus, delirium, coma and convulsions, depending on the substance and method of administration.

Opioid overdose

The use of opioids in amounts that produce acute adverse physical or mental effects. Deliberate overdose is a common method of suicide. In absolute numbers, overdoses of licit opioids tend to be more common than those of illicit opioids. Overdose may produce transient or lasting effects, or death; the lethal dose of a particular opioid varies with the individual and with circumstances.

Opioid-use disorders

A group of conditions associated with the use of opioids. In ICD-I0, section F11.0–9 ("Mental and behavioural disorders due to psychoactive substance use (opioids)") contains a wide variety of disorders of different severity and clinical form, all having in common the use of opioids, which may or may not have been medically prescribed. The clinical states that may occur include acute intoxication, harmful use, dependence syndrome, withdrawal syndrome (or withdrawal state), withdrawal state with delirium, psychotic disorder, late-onset psychotic disorder and amnesic syndrome.

Opioid withdrawal syndrome

Over time, morphine and its analogues induce tolerance and neuroadaptive changes that are responsible for rebound hyperexcitability when the drug is withdrawn. The withdrawal syndrome includes craving, anxiety, dysphoria, yawning, sweating, piloerection (gooseflesh), lacrimation (excessive tear formation), rhinorrhoea (running nose), insomnia, nausea or vomiting, diarrhoea, cramps, muscle aches and fever. With short-acting drugs, such as morphine or heroin, withdrawal symptoms may appear within 8–12 hours of the last dose of the drug, reach a peak at 48–72 hours, and clear after 7–10 days. With longer acting drugs, such as methadone, onset of withdrawal symptoms may not occur until 1–3 days after the last dose; symptoms peak between the third and eighth day and may persist for several weeks, but are generally milder than those that follow morphine or heroin withdrawal after equivalent doses.

Psychosocial intervention

Any non-pharmacological intervention carried out in a therapeutic context at an individual, family or group level. Psychosocial interventions may include structured, professionally administered interventions (e.g. cognitive behaviour therapy or insight oriented psychotherapy) or non-professional interventions (e.g. self-help groups and non-pharmacological interventions from traditional healers).

Psychotropic substance

Psychotropic substances are the substances, natural or synthetic, or any natural material in Schedules I, II, III or IV of the Convention on Psychotropic Substances, 1971, (see above). Among others, buprenorphine and benzodiazepines are psychotropic substances.

Single Convention on Narcotic Drugs, 1961

The Single Convention on Narcotic Drugs, 1961 (as amended by the 1972 Protocol) is the main international drug control treaty. Replacing a number of previous conventions, it aims to limit the cultivation, production, manufacture and use of narcotic drugs to medical and scientific purposes, while ensuring their availability for such purposes. The convention lists a number of narcotic drugs, and outlines the responsibilities of parties with regard to the production, manufacture, distribution and use of these drugs in their countries. The INCB, which submits its reports to ECOSOC through the CND, is responsible for monitoring the compliance of governments with the provisions of this treaty. Methadone is listed in the Single Convention on Narcotic Drugs, 1961.

Tolerance

A decrease in response to a drug dose that occurs with continued use. If an individual is tolerant to a drug, increased doses are required to achieve the effects originally produced by lower doses. Both physiological and psychosocial factors may contribute to the development of tolerance. Physiological factors include metabolic and functional tolerance. In metabolic tolerance, the body can eliminate the substance more readily, because the substance is metabolized at an increased rate. In functional tolerance, the central nervous system is less sensitive to the substance. An example of a psychosocial factor contributing to tolerance is behavioural tolerance, where learning or altered environmental constraints change the effect of the drug. Acute tolerance refers to rapid, temporary accommodation to the effect of a substance following a single dose. Reverse tolerance, also known as sensitization, refers to a condition where the response to a substance increases with repeated use. Tolerance is one of the criteria of the dependence syndrome.

Withdrawal syndrome (abstinence syndrome, withdrawal reaction, withdrawal state)

A group of symptoms of variable clustering and degree of severity that occur on cessation or reduction of use of a psychoactive substance that has been taken repeatedly, usually for a prolonged period or in high doses (ICD-10 code F1x.3). Withdrawal syndrome may be accompanied by signs of physiological disturbance. It is one of the indicators of dependence syndrome, and is the defining characteristic of the psychopharmacological definition of dependence.

The onset and course of withdrawal syndrome are time limited and relate to the type of substance and dose being taken immediately before cessation or reduction of use. Typically, the features of withdrawal syndrome are the opposite of acute intoxication.

Opioid withdrawal is accompanied by rhinorrhoea (running nose), lacrimation (excessive tear formation), aching muscles, chills, piloerection (gooseflesh) and, after 24–48 hours, muscle and abdominal cramps. Drug-seeking behaviour is prominent and continues after the physical symptoms have abated.

References

1. Economic and Social Council (2004). *ECOSOC resolution 2004/40*, http://www.un.org/docs/ecosoc/documents/2004/resolutions/eres2004-40.pdf (accessed 1/2/2008).

2. United Nations Office on Drugs and Crime (2007). *World Drug Report*.

3. Hser YI, Hoffman V, Grella CE and Anglin MD (2001). A 33-year follow-up of narcotics addicts. *Archives of General Psychiatry*, 58(5):503-508.

4. Mark TL, Woody GE, Juday T and Kleber HD (2001). The economic costs of heroin addiction in the United States. *Drug Alcohol Dependence*, 61(2):195-206.

5. UNAIDS (Joint United Nations Programme on HIV/AIDS) (2006). *Report on the global AIDS epidemic*. Geneva, Switzerland. http://www.unaids.org/en/KnowledgeCentre/HIVData/GlobalReport/2006/ (Accessed 14 July 2008).

6. Piot P and Coll Seck AM (2001). International response to the HIV/AIDS epidemic: planning for success. *Bulletin of the World Health Organization*, 79(12):1106-1112.

7. World Health Organization (2004) *WHO/UNODC/UNAIDS position paper. Substitution maintenance therapy in the management of opioid dependence and HIV/AIDS prevention*. Geneva, WHO.

8. World Health Organization (2007). *WHO Model List of Essential Medicines*. Geneva, World Health Organization. Available from URL: http://www.who.int/medicines.

9. World Health Organization (2004). *Neuroscience of psychoactive substance use and dependence*. Geneva, WHO.

10. World Health Organization (1996). *WHO Expert Committee on Drug Dependence*. Geneva, Switzerland, 13th report, WHO technical report series 873. http://whqlibdoc.who.int/trs/WHO_TRS_873.pdf (Accessed 9 July 2008)

11. World Health Organization (2006). *Basic Principles for Treatment and Psychosocial Support of Drug Dependent People Living with HIV/AIDS*. Geneva, WHO.

12. World Health Organization (2002). *Guidelines for WHO Guidelines, Global Programme on Evidence for Health Policy*. http://libdoc.who.int/hq/2003/EIP_GPE_EQC_2003_1.pdf (Accessed 9 July 2008).

13. Atkins D, Eccles M, Flottorp S, Guyatt GH, Henry D, Hill S, Liberati A, O'Connell D, Oxman AD, Phillips B, Schunemann H, Edejer TT, Vist GE and Williams JW, Jr. (2004). Systems for grading the quality of evidence and the strength of recommendations I: critical appraisal of existing approaches The GRADE Working Group. *BMC Health Services Research*, 4(1):38.

14. World Health Organization (2007). *International Classification of Diseases, 10th edition (ICD-10)*. http://www.who.int/classifications/apps/icd/icd10online/ (Accessed 2008 9 July).

15. Volkow ND and Li TK (2004). Drug addiction: the neurobiology of behaviour gone awry. *Nature Reviews. Neuroscience*. 5(12):963-970.

16. Ballantyne JC and LaForge KS (2007). Opioid dependence and addiction during opioid treatment of chronic pain. *Pain*. 129(3):235-255.

17. Yaksh TL (1984). Multiple opioid receptor systems in brain and spinal cord: Part I. *European Journal of Anaesthesiology*. 1(2):171-199.

18. Yaksh TL (1984). Multiple opioid receptor systems in brain and spinal cord: Part 2. *European Journal of Anaesthesiology*. 1(3):201-243.

19. Bodnar RJ and Klein GE (2006). Endogenous opiates and behavior: 2005. *Peptides*, 27(12):3391-3478.

20. Johnson SW and North RA (1992). Opioids excite dopamine neurons by hyperpolarization of local interneurons. *Journal of Neuroscience*. 12(2):483-488.

21. Bonci A and Williams JT (1997). Increased probability of GABA release during withdrawal from morphine. *Journal of Neuroscience*. 17(2):796-803.

22. Cami J and Farre M (2003). Drug addiction. *New England Journal of Medicine*. 349(10):975-986.

23. Nestler EJ, Berhow MT and Brodkin ES (1996). Molecular mechanisms of drug addiction: adaptations in signal transduction pathways. *Molecular Psychiatry*. 1(3):190-199.

24. Hyman SE and Malenka RC (2001). Addiction and the brain: the neurobiology of compulsion and its persistence. *Nature Reviews. Neuroscience*. 2(10):695-703.

25. Williams JT, Christie MJ and Manzoni O (2001). Cellular and synaptic adaptations mediating opioid dependence. *Physiological Reviews*. 81(1):299-343.

26. Kieffer BL and Evans CJ (2002). Opioid tolerance-in search of the holy grail. *Cell*, 108(5):587-590.

27. US Census Bureau (2004). *The AIDS Pandemic in the 21st Century*. International Population Reports. Washington, DC, US Government Printing Office, WP/02-2.

28. Centers for Disease Control (1998). *Mortality and Morbidity Weekly Report.*, 47(RR-19).

29. Hulse GK, English DR, Milne E and Holman CD (1999). The quantification of mortality resulting from the regular use of illicit opiates. *Addiction*. 94(2):221-229.

30. Darke S and Ross J (2002). Suicide among heroin users: rates, risk factors and methods. *Addiction*. 97(11):1383-1394.

31. Vlahov D, Wang CL, Galai N, Bareta J, Mehta SH, Strathdee SA and Nelson KE (2004). Mortality risk among new onset injection drug users. *Addiction*. 99(8):946-954.

32. Goldstein A and Herrera J (1995). Heroin addicts and methadone treatment in Albuquerque: a 22-year follow-up. *Drug and Alcohol Dependence*. 40(2):139-150.

33. Bargagli AM, Sperati A, Davoli M, Forastiere F and Perucci CA (2001). Mortality among problem drug users in Rome: an 18-year follow-up study, 1980–97. *Addiction*. 96(10):1455-1463.

34. Stein MD, Mulvey KP, Plough A and Samet JH (1998). The functioning and well being of persons who seek treatment for drug and alcohol use. *J Subst Abuse*, 10(1):75-84.

35. Ross J, Teesson M, Darke S, Lynskey M, Ali R, Ritter A and Cooke R (2005). The characteristics of heroin users entering treatment: findings from the Australian treatment outcome study (ATOS). *Drug and Alcohol Review*. 24(5):411-418.

36. Collins DJ and Lapsley HM (1996). *The social costs of drug abuse in Australia in 1988 and 1992*. Canberra, Australia.

37. Xie X, Rehm J, Single E, Robson L and Paul J (1998). The economic costs of Illicit drug use in Ontario, 1992. *electronic Health Economics letters*, 2(1):8-14.

38. Clark, N., Gospodarevskaya, E., Harris, A. & Ritter, A. *Estimating the Cost of Heroin Use in Victoria*. Report to the Premier's Drug Prevention Council. Melbourne: Department of Human Services 2003. Available online at URL: http://www.druginfo.adf.org.au/hidden_articles/estimating_the_cost_of_heroin_1.html39.

39. Darke S, Ross J, Mills KL, Williamson A, Havard A and Teesson M (2007). Patterns of sustained heroin abstinence amongst long-term, dependent heroin users: 36 months findings from the Australian Treatment Outcome Study (ATOS). *Addictive Behaviors*. 32(9):1897-1906.

40. Maddux JF and Desmond DP (1992). Methadone maintenance and recovery from opioid dependence. *American Journal of Drug and Alcohol Abuse*. 18(1):63-74.

41. Flynn PM, Joe GW, Broome KM, Simpson DD and Brown BS (2003). Recovery from opioid addiction in DATOS. *Journal of Substance Abuse Treatment*, 25(3):177-186.

42. Hser YI (2007). Predicting long-term stable recovery from heroin addiction: findings from a 33-year follow-up study. *Journal of Addictive Diseases*, 26(1):51-60.

43. Teesson M, Ross J, Darke S, Lynskey M, Ali R, Ritter A and Cooke R (2006). One year outcomes for heroin dependence: findings from the Australian Treatment Outcome Study (ATOS). *Drug & Alcohol Dependence*, 83(2):174-180.

44. Gandhi DH, Jaffe JH, McNary S, Kavanagh GJ, Hayes M and Currens M (2003). Short-term outcomes after brief ambulatory opioid detoxification with buprenorphine in young heroin users. *Addiction*. 98(4):453-462.

45. Hser YI, Anglin MD and Fletcher B (1998). Comparative treatment effectiveness. Effects of program modality and client drug dependence history on drug use reduction. *Journal of Substance Abuse Treatment*, 15(6):513-523.

46. Calsyn DA, Malcy JA and Saxon AJ (2006). Slow tapering from methadone maintenance in a program encouraging indefinite maintenance. *Journal of Substance Abuse Treatment*, 30(2):159-163.

47. Lenne M, Lintzeris N, Breen C, Harris S, Hawken L, Mattick R and Ritter A (2001). Withdrawal from methadone maintenance treatment: prognosis and

participant perspectives. *Australian & New Zealand Journal of Public Health*, 25(2):121-125.

48. Hiltunen AJ and Eklund C (2002). Withdrawal from methadone maintenance treatment. Reasons for not trying to quit methadone. *European Addiction Research*, 8(1):38-44.

49. World Health Organization (2006). *Constitution of the World Health Organization*. Geneva, Basic Documents, 45th edition, Supplement October 2006. http://www.who.int/governance/eb/who_constitution_en.pdf (Accessed 9 July 2008).

50. World Health Organization (1986). www.who.int/hpr/NPH/docs/ottawa_charter_hp.pdf (accessed 12 December, 2008).

51. Hall WD, Ross JE, Lynskey MT, Law MG and Degenhardt LJ (2000). How many dependent heroin users are there in Australia? *Medical Journal of Australia*. 173(10):528-531.

52. World Health Organization (1993). WHO Expert Committee on Drug Dependence, Twenty-eighth Report. *WHO Technical Report Series*, No. 836.

53. Reilly D, Scantleton J and Didcott P (2002). Magistrates' Early Referral into Treatment (MERIT): preliminary findings of a 12-month court diversion trial for drug offenders. *Drug and Alcohol Review*. 21(4):393-396.

54. Fielding JE, Tye G, Ogawa PL, Imam IJ and Long AM (2002). Los Angeles County drug court programs: initial results. *Journal of Substance Abuse Treatment*. 23(3):217-224.

55. Britton B (1994). The privatization of methadone maintenance; changes in risk behavior associated with cost related detoxification. *Addiction Research*, 2(2):171-181.

56. McCollister K and French M (2003). The relative contribution of outcome domains in the total economic benefit of addiction interventions: a review of first findings. *Addiction*. 98:1647–1659.

57. French M and Drummond M (2005). A research agenda for economic evaluation of substance abuse services. *Journal of Substance Abuse Treatment*, 29:125-137.

58. French M and Martin R (1996). The Costs of Drug Abuse Consequences: A Summary of Research Findings. *Journal of Substance Abuse Treatment*, 13(6):453-466.

59. Choi B, Robson L and Single E (1997). Estimating the economic costs of the abuse of tobacco, alcohol and illicit drugs: a review of methodologies and Canadian data sources. *Chronic Diseases in Canada*, 18(4):149-165.

60. Cartwright WS (2000). Cost-benefit analysis of drug treatment services: review of the literature. *Journal of Mental Health Policy and Economics*, 3:11-26.

61. Hall W, Doran C, Degenhardt L and Shepard D (2006). Illicit Opioid Use. In: Musgrove P, ed. *Disease control priorities in developing countries*. New York, Oxford University Press, 2, 907-932.

62. Simoens S, Ludbrook A, Matheson C and Bond C (2006). Pharmaco-economics of community maintenance for opiate dependence: a review of evidence and methodology. *Drug and Alcohol Dependence*. 84(1):28-39.

63. Simoens S, Matheson C, Inkster K, Ludbrook A and Bond C (2002). *The effectiveness of treatment for drug users: An international systematic review of the evidence*. Edinburgh, Scottish Executive Drug Misuse Research Programme

64. World Health Organization (2008). *Choosing Interventions that are Cost Effective: Cost-it*. http://www.who.int/choice/toolkit/cost_it/en/ (Accessed 2008 16 July).

65. Dole VP and Nyswander M (1965). A medical treatment for diacetylmorphine (heroin) addiction. *Journal of the American Medical Association*, 193:80-84.

66. Dole V, Robinson J and Orraca J (1969). Methadone treatment of randomly selected criminal addicts. *New Engand Journal of Medicine*, 280:1372-1375.

67. Dole VP (1971). *Methadone maintenance treatment for 25000 addicts*. Journal of the American Medical Association, 215:1131-1134.

68. Lintzeris N, Ritter A, Panjari M, Clark N, Kutin J and Bammer G (2004). Implementing buprenorphine treatment in community settings in Australia: experiences from the Buprenorphine Implementation Trial. *American Journal of Addiction*. 13 Suppl 1:S29-41.

69. Alford DP, LaBelle CT, Richardson JM, O'Connell JJ, Hohl CA, Cheng DM and Samet JH (2007). Treating homeless opioid dependent patients with buprenorphine in an office-based setting. *Journal of General Internal Medicine*. 22(2):171-176.

70. Fiellin DA, O'Connor PG, Chawarski M, Pakes JP, Pantalon MV and Schottenfeld RS (2001). Methadone maintenance in primary care: a randomized controlled trial. *Jama.* 286(14):1724-1731.

71. Bell J, Dru A, Fischer B, Levit S and Sarfraz MA (2002). Substitution therapy for heroin addiction. *Substance Use and Misuse.* 37(8-10):1149-1178.

72. Gibson AE, Doran CM, Bell JR, Ryan A and Lintzeris N (2003). A comparison of buprenorphine treatment in clinic and primary care settings: a randomised trial. *Medical Journal of Australia.* 179(1):38-42.

73. Vignau J, Boissonnas A, Tignol J, Millot Y and Mucchielli A (2003). [French nationwide survey of abstinence-oriented treatments in opiate-addicted patients. Results at 12 months]. *Annales de Médecine Interne (Paris).* 154 Spec No 2:S23-32.

74. World Health Organization (2007). *Health in prisons: A WHO guide to the essentials in prison health.* http://www.euro.who.int/document/e90174.pdf (Accessed 09 July 2008).

75. United Nations General Assembly (1966). International Covenant on Economic, Social and Cultural Rights. *http://www.unhchr.ch/html/menu3/b/a_cescr.htm (accessed 2008 1 March)*, resolution 2200A (XXI).

76. World Health Organization (2005). *WHO Resource Book on Mental Health, Human Rights and Legislation.* Geneva, WHO.

77. Kornor H and Waal H (2005). From opioid maintenance to abstinence: a literature review. *Drug and Alcohol Review.* 24(3):267-274.

78. Piper TM, Rudenstine S, Stancliff S, Sherman S, Nandi V, Clear A and Galea S (2007). Overdose prevention for injection drug users: lessons learned from naloxone training and distribution programs in New York City. *Harm Reduction Journal.* 4:3.

79. Seal KH, Thawley R, Gee L, Bamberger J, Kral AH, Ciccarone D, Downing M and Edlin BR (2005). Naloxone distribution and cardiopulmonary resuscitation training for injection drug users to prevent heroin overdose death: a pilot intervention study. *Journal of Urban Health.* 82(2):303-311.

80. Fry C, Dietze P and Crofts N (2000). Naloxone distribution: remembering hepatitis C transmission as an issue. *Addiction.* 95(12):1865-1866.

81. Wang H, He G, Li X, Yang A, Chen X, Fennie KP and Williams AB (2008). Self-Reported Adherence to Antiretroviral Treatment among HIV-Infected People in Central China. *AIDS Patient Care STDS.* 22(1): 71-80.

82. Smith-Rohrberg D, Mezger J, Walton M, Bruce RD and Altice FL (2006). Impact of enhanced services on virologic outcomes in a directly administered antiretroviral therapy trial for HIV-infected drug users. *Journal of the Acquired Immunodeficiency Syndrome.* 43 Suppl 1:S48-53.

83. Lucas GM, Gebo KA, Chaisson RE and Moore RD (2002). Longitudinal assessment of the effects of drug and alcohol abuse on HIV-1 treatment outcomes in an urban clinic. *Aids.* 16(5):767-774.

84. van Beek I (2007). Case study: accessible primary health care – a foundation to improve health outcomes for people who inject drugs. *International Journal of Drug Policy.* 18(4):329-332.

85. Krook AL, Stokka D, Heger B and Nygaard E (2007). Hepatitis C treatment of opioid dependants receiving maintenance treatment: results of a Norwegian pilot study. *European Addiction Research.* 13(4):216-221.

86. Sylvestre DL and Clements BJ (2007). Adherence to hepatitis C treatment in recovering heroin users maintained on methadone. *European Journal of Gastroenterology and Hepatology.* 19(9):741-747.

87. Edlin BR, Kresina TF, Raymond DB, Carden MR, Gourevitch MN, Rich JD, Cheever LW and Cargill VA (2005). Overcoming barriers to prevention, care, and treatment of hepatitis C in illicit drug users. *Clinical Infectious Disease.* 40 Suppl 5:S276-285.

88. Umbricht-Schneiter A, Ginn DH, Pabst KM and Bigelow GE (1994). Providing medical care to methadone clinic patients: referral vs on-site care. *American Journal of Public Health.* 84(2):207-210.

89. Weisner C, Mertens J, Parthasarathy S, Moore C and Lu Y (2001). Integrating primary medical care with addiction treatment: a randomized controlled trial. *Jama.* 286(14):1715-1723.

90. Willenbring ML and Olson DH (1999). A randomized trial of integrated outpatient treatment for medically ill alcoholic men. *Archives of Internal Medicine.* 159(16):1946-1952.

91. Scholten JN, Driver CR, Munsiff SS, Kaye K, Rubino MA, Gourevitch MN, Trim C, Amofa J, Seewald R, Highley E and Fujiwara PI (2003). Effectiveness of isoniazid treatment for latent tuberculosis infection among human immunodeficiency virus (HIV)-infected and HIV-uninfected injection drug users in methadone programs. *Clinical Infectious Disease.* 37(12):1686-1692.

92. Gourevitch MN, Selwyn PA, Davenny K, Buono D, Schoenbaum EE, Klein RS and Friedland GH (1993). Effects of HIV infection on the serologic manifestations and response to treatment of syphilis in intravenous drug users. *Annals of Internal Medicine*. 118(5):350-355.

93. O'Connor PG, Molde S, Henry S, Shockcor WT and Schottenfeld RS (1992). Human immunodeficiency virus infection in intravenous drug users: a model for primary care. *American Journal of Medicine*. 93(4):382-386.

94. Newman RG (1994). More on methadone treatment. *American Journal of Public Health*. 84(11):1854.

95. World Health Organization (2004). *Weekly Epidemiological Record*, 28(79):253–264.

96. Altice FL, Bruce RD, Walton MR and Buitrago MI (2005). Adherence to hepatitis B virus vaccination at syringe exchange sites. *Journal of Urban Health*. 82(1):151-161.

97. Christensen PB, Fisker N, Krarup HB, Liebert E, Jaroslavtsev N, Christensen K and Georgsen J (2004). Hepatitis B vaccination in prison with a 3-week schedule is more efficient than the standard 6-month schedule. *Vaccine*. 22(29-30):3897-3901.

98. Macdonald V, Dore GJ, Amin J and van Beek I (2007). Predictors of completion of a hepatitis B vaccination schedule in attendees at a primary health care centre. *Sex Health*. 4(1):27-30.

99. Okruhlica L and Klempova D (2002). Hodnocení programu vakcinace proti hepatitide typu B u uživatelú drog v Bratislave (Evaluation of a Hepatitis B Vaccination Programme among Drug Users in Bratislava). *Adiktologie*, 2:11-18.

100. Quaglio G, Talamini G, Lugoboni F, Lechi A, Venturini L, Jarlais D and Mezzelani P (2003). Compliance with hepatitis B vaccination in 1175 heroin users and risk factors associated with lack of vaccine response. *Addiction*. 97(12):1611-1613.

101. Mattos A, Gomes E, Tovo C, Alexandre C and Remião J (2004). Hepatitis B vaccine efficacy in patients with chronic liver disease by hepatitis C virus. *Arq Gastroenterol*. 41(3):180-184.

102. World Health Organization (2000). *Weekly Epidemiological Record*, 5(75):37-44.

103. World Health Organization (2008). *WHO collaborative research project on drug dependence treatment and HIV/AIDS*. http://www.who.int/substance_abuse/activities/treatment_HIV/en/index.html (Accessed 12 December 2008).

104. Williams JT, Christie MJ and Manzoni O (2001). Cellular and synaptic adaptations mediating opioid dependence. *Physiological Reviews*, 81(1):299-343.

105. Mattick RP, Breen C, Kimber J and Davoli M (in press). Methadone maintenance therapy versus no opioid replacement therapy for opioid dependence. *Cochrane Database Systematic Review*.

106. Newman RG and Whitehill WB (1979). Double-blind comparison of methadone and placebo maintenance treatments of narcotic addicts in Hong Kong. *Lancet*. 2(8141):485-488.

107. Vanichseni S, Wongsuwan B, Choopanya K and Wongpanich K (1991). A controlled trial of methadone maintenance in a population of intravenous drug users in Bangkok: implications for prevention of HIV. *International Journal of Addiction*. 26(12):1313-1320.

108. Strain EC, Stitzer ML, Liebson IA and Bigelow GE (1993). Dose-response effects of methadone in the treatment of opioid dependence. *Annals of Internal Medicine*. 119(1):23-27.

109. Johnson RE, Eissenberg T, Stitzer ML, Strain EC, Liebson IA and Bigelow GE (1995). A placebo controlled clinical trial of buprenorphine as a treatment for opioid dependence. *Drug and Alcohol Dependence*. 40(1):17-25.

110. Ling W, Charuvastra C, Collins JF, Batki S, Brown LS, Jr, Kintaudi P, Wesson DR, McNicholas L, Tusel DJ, Malkerneker U, Renner JA, Jr, Santos E, Casadonte P, Fye C, Stine S, Wang RI and Segal D (1998). Buprenorphine maintenance treatment of opiate dependence: a multicenter, randomized clinical trial. *Addiction*. 93(4):475-486.

111. Caplehorn JRM and Drummer OH (1999). Mortality associated with New South Wales methadone programs in 1994: lives lost and saved. *Medical Journal of Australia*, 170:104-109.

112. Lawrinson P, Ali R, Uchtenhagen A and Newcombe D (2009). *The WHO Collaborative Study on Substitution Therapy of Opioid Dependence and HIV/AIDS*. Geneva. http://www.who.int/substance_abuse/en/index.html.

113. Moore TJ, Ritter A and Caulkins JP (2007). The costs and consequences of three policy options for reducing heroin dependency. *Drug and Alcohol Review*. 26(4):369-378.

114. Zarkin GA, Dunlap LJ, Hicks KA and Mamo D (2005). Benefits and costs of methadone treatment: results from a lifetime simulation model. *Health Economics.* 14(11):1133-1150.

115. Barnett PG (1999). The cost-effectiveness of methadone maintenance as a health care intervention. *Addiction.* 94(4):479-488.

116. Hall WD, Doran CM, Degenhardt LJ and Shepard D (2006). Illicit Opiate Abuse. In: Department of Mental Health and Substance Abuse, ed. *Disease Control Priorities related to Mental, Neurological, Developmental and Substance Abuse Disorders.* Geneva, World Health Organization, 77-100.

117. Bell J, Digiusto E and Byth K (1992). Who should receive methadone maintenance? *British Journal of Addiction.* 87(5):689-694.

118. Mattick RP, Kimber J, Breen C and Davoli M (2004). Buprenorphine maintenance versus placebo or methadone maintenance for opioid dependence. *Cochrane Database Systematic Review.*(3):CD002207.

119. Auriacombe M, Fatseas M, Dubernet J, Daulouede JP and Tignol J (2004). French field experience with buprenorphine. *American Journal of Addiction.* 13 Suppl 1:S17-28.

120. Auriacombe M, Franques P and Tignol J (2001). Deaths attributable to methadone vs buprenorphine in France. *Jama.* 285(1):45.

121. Kintz P (2002). A new series of 13 buprenorphine-related deaths. *Clinical Biochemistry.* 35(7):513-516.

122. Kintz P (2001). Deaths involving buprenorphine: a compendium of French cases. *Forensic Science International.* 121(1-2):65-69.

123. Anonymous (2006). Buprenorphine replacement therapy: a confirmed benefit. *Prescrire International.* 15(82):64-70.

124. Bargagli AM, Sperati A, Davoli M, Forastiere F and Perucci CA (2001). Mortality among problem drug users in Rome: an 18-year follow-up study, 1980-97. *Addiction.* 96(10):1455-1463.

125. Petitjean S, Stohler R, Deglon JJ, Livoti S, Waldvogel D, Uehlinger C and Ladewig D (2001). Double-blind randomized trial of buprenorphine and methadone in opiate dependence. *Drug and Alcohol Dependence.* 62(1):97-104.

126. Soyka M, Hock B, Kagerer S, Lehnert R, Limmer C and Kuefner H (2005). Less impairment on one portion of a driving-relevant psychomotor battery in buprenorphine-maintained than in methadone-maintained patients: results of a randomized clinical trial. *Journal of Clinical Psychopharmacology.* 25(5):490-493.

127. Lenné M, Dietze P, Rumbold GR, Redman JR and Triggs TJ (2003). The effects of the opioid pharmacotherapies methadone, LAAM and buprenorphine, alone and in combination with alcohol, on simulated driving. *Drug and Alcohol Dependence.* 72(3):271-278.

128. Jenkinson RA, Clark NC, Fry CL and Dobbin M (2005). Buprenorphine diversion and injection in Melbourne, Australia: an emerging issue? *Addiction.* 100(2):197-205.

129. Fanoe S, Hvidt C, Ege P and Jensen GB (2007). Syncope and QT prolongation among patients treated with methadone for heroin dependence in the city of Copenhagen. *Heart.* 93(9):1051-5.

130. Anonymous (2005). Torsades de pointes with methadone. *Prescrire International.* 14(76):61-62.

131. Krantz MJ, Garcia JA and Mehler PS (2005). Effects of buprenorphine on cardiac repolarization in a patient with methadone-related torsade de pointes. *Pharmacotherapy.* 25(4):611-614.

132. Baker JR, Best AM, Pade PA and McCance-Katz EF (2006). Effect of buprenorphine and antiretroviral agents on the QT interval in opioid-dependent patients. *Annals of Pharmacotherapy.* 40(3):392-396.

133. Dyer KR and White JM (1997). Patterns of symptom complaints in methadone maintenance patients. *Addiction.* 92(11):1445-1455.

134. Caplehorn JR, Bell J, Kleinbaum DG and Gebski VJ (1993). Methadone dose and heroin use during maintenance treatment. *Addiction.* 88(1):119-124.

135. D'Ippoliti D, Davoli M, Perucci CA, Pasqualini F and Bargagli AM (1998). Retention in treatment of heroin users in Italy: The role of treatment type and of methadone maintenance dosage. *Drug and Alcohol Dependence.* 52(2):167-171.

136. Maxwell S and Shinderman M (1999). Optimizing response to methadone maintenance treatment: use of higher- dose methadone. *Journal of Psychoactive Drugs.* 31(2):95-102.

137. Strain EC, Stitzer ML, Liebson IA and Bigelow GE (1993). Methadone dose and treatment outcome. *Drug and Alcohol Dependence.* 33(2):105-117.

138. Hartel DM, Schoenbaum EE, Selwyn PA, Kline J, Davenny K, Klein RS and Friedland GH (1995). Heroin use during methadone maintenance treatment: the importance of methadone dose and cocaine use. *American Journal of Public Health.* 85(1):83-88.

139. Gerra G, Ferri M, Polidori E, Santoro G, Zaimovic A and Sternieri E (2003). Long-term methadone maintenance effectiveness: psychosocial and pharmacological variables. *Journal of Substance Abuse Treatment.* 25(1):1-8.

140. Faggiano F, Vigna-Taglianti F, Versino E and Lemma P (2003). Methadone maintenance at different dosages for opioid dependence. *Cochrane Database Systematic Review.* (3):CD002208.

141. Kosten TR, Schottenfeld R, Ziedonis D and Falcioni J (1993). Buprenorphine versus methadone maintenance for opioid dependence. *Journal of Nervous and Mental Disease.* 181(6):358-364.

142. Ahmadi J (2003). Methadone versus buprenorphine maintenance for the treatment of heroin-dependent outpatients. *Journal of Substance Abuse Treatment.* 24(3):217-220.

143. Schottenfeld RS, Pakes JR, Oliveto A, Ziedonis D and Kosten TR (1997). Buprenorphine vs methadone maintenance treatment for concurrent opioid dependence and cocaine abuse [see comments]. *Archives of General Psychiatry.* 54(8):713-720.

144. Montoya ID, Gorelick DA, Preston KL, Schroeder JR, Umbricht A, Cheskin LJ, Lange WR, Contoreggi C, Johnson RE and Fudala PJ (2004). Randomized trial of buprenorphine for treatment of concurrent opiate and cocaine dependence. *Clinical Pharmacology and Therapeutics.* 75(1):34-48.

145. Walsh SL, Preston KL, Bigelow GE and Stitzer ML (1995). Acute administration of buprenorphine in humans: partial agonist and blockade effects. *Journal of Pharmacology and Experimental Therapeutics.* 274(1):361-372.

146. Comer SD, Collins ED and Fischman MW (2001). Buprenorphine sublingual tablets: effects on IV heroin self- administration by humans. *Psychopharmacology (Berl).* 154(1):28-37.

147. Greenwald MK, Johanson CE and Schuster CR (1999). Opioid reinforcement in heroin-dependent volunteers during outpatient buprenorphine maintenance. *Drug and Alcohol Dependence.* 56(3):191-203.

148. Greenwald MK, Schuh KJ, Hopper JA, Schuster CR and Johanson CE (2002). Effects of buprenorphine sublingual tablet maintenance on opioid drug-seeking behavior by humans. *Psychopharmacology (Berl).* 160(4):344-352.

149. Schottenfeld RS, Pakes J, Zidenois D and Kosten TR (1993). Buprenorphine: Dose-related effects on cocaine and opioid use in cocaine-abusing opioid dependent humans. *Biological Psychiatry*, 34:66-74.

150. Strain EC, Walsh SL and Bigelow GE (2002). Blockade of hydromorphone effects by buprenorphine/naloxone and buprenorphine. *Psychopharmacology (Berl).* 159(2):161-166.

151. Winstock AR, Lea T and Sheridan J (2008). Prevalence of diversion and injection of methadone and buprenorphine among clients receiving opioid treatment at community pharmacies in New South Wales, Australia. *International Journal of Drug Policy.* 19(6):450-8.

152. Vlahov D, O'Driscoll P, Mehta SH, Ompad DC, Gern R, Galai N and Kirk GD (2007). Risk factors for methadone outside treatment programs: implications for HIV treatment among injection drug users. *Addiction.* 102(5):771-777.

153. Shields LB, Hunsaker Iii JC, Corey TS, Ward MK and Stewart D (2007). Methadone toxicity fatalities: a review of medical examiner cases in a large metropolitan area. *Journal of Forensic Science.* 52(6):1389-1395.

154. Gunderson EW and Fiellin DA (2008). Office-Based Maintenance Treatment of Opioid Dependence : How Does it Compare With Traditional Approaches? *CNS Drugs*, 22(2):99-111.

155. Kraft MK, Rothbard AB, Hadley TR, McLellan AT and Asch DA (1997). Are supplementary services provided during methadone maintenance really cost-effective? *American Journal of Psychiatry.* 154(9):1214-1219.

156. McLellan AT, Arndt IO, Metzger DS, Woody GE and O'Brien CP (1993). The effects of psychosocial services in substance abuse treatment. *Jama.* 269(15):1953-1959.

157. Avants SK, Margolin A, Sindelar JL, Rounsaville BJ, Schottenfeld R, Stine S, Cooney NL, Rosenheck RA, Li SH and Kosten TR (1999). Day treatment versus enhanced standard methadone services for opioid-dependent patients: a comparison of clinical efficacy and cost. *American Journal of Psychiatry.* 156(1):27-33.

158. Shanahan MD, Doran CM, Digiusto E, Bell J, Lintzeris N, White J, Ali R, Saunders JB, Mattick RP and Gilmour S (2006). A cost-effectiveness analysis

of heroin detoxification methods in the Australian National Evaluation of Pharmacotherapies for Opioid Dependence (NEPOD). *Addictive Behaviors.* 31(3):371-387.

159. Gowing L, Ali R and White J (2004). Buprenorphine for the management of opioid withdrawal. *Cochrane Database Systematic Review.* (4):CD002025.

160. Gowing L, Ali R and White J (2006). Opioid antagonists with minimal sedation for opioid withdrawal. *Cochrane Database Systematic Review.* (1):CD002021.

161. Gowing L, Ali R and White J (2006). Opioid antagonists under heavy sedation or anaesthesia for opioid withdrawal. *Cochrane Database Systematic Review.* (2):CD002022.

162. McGregor C, Ali R, White JM, Thomas P and Gowing L (2002). A comparison of antagonist-precipitated withdrawal under anesthesia to standard inpatient withdrawal as a precursor to maintenance naltrexone treatment in heroin users: outcomes at 6 and 12 months. *Drug and Alcohol Dependence.* 68(1):5-14.

163. Collins ED, Kleber HD, Whittington RA and Heitler NE (2005). Anesthesia-assisted vs buprenorphine- or clonidine-assisted heroin detoxification and naltrexone induction: a randomized trial. *Jama.* 294(8):903-913.

164. Seoane A, Carrasco G, Cabre L, Puiggros A, Hernandez E, Alvarez M, Costa J, Molina R and Sobrepere G (1997). Efficacy and safety of two new methods of rapid intravenous detoxification in heroin addicts previously treated without success [published erratum appears in Br J Psychiatry 1997 Dec;171:588]. *British Journal of Psychiatry.* 171:340-345.

165. De Jong CA, Laheij RJ and Krabbe PF (2005). General anaesthesia does not improve outcome in opioid antagonist detoxification treatment: a randomized controlled trial. *Addiction.* 100(2):206-215.

166. Hamilton RJ, Olmedo RE, Shah S, Hung OL, Howland MA, Perrone J, Nelson LS, Lewin NL and Hoffman RS (2002). Complications of ultrarapid opioid detoxification with subcutaneous naltrexone pellets.*Academic Emergency Medicine.* 9(1):63-68.

167. Kaye AD, Gevirtz C, Bosscher HA, Duke JB, Frost EA, Richards TA and Fields AM (2003). Ultrarapid opiate detoxification: a review. *Canadian Journal of Anaesthesiology.* 50(7):663-671.

168. Day E, Ison J and Strang J (2005). Inpatient versus other settings for detoxification for opioid dependence. *Cochrane Database Systematic Review.* (2):CD004580.

169. Amato L, Minozzi S, Davoli M, Vecchi S, Ferri M and Mayet S (2004). Psychosocial and pharmacological treatments versus pharmacological treatments for opioid detoxification. *Cochrane Database Systematic Review.*(4):CD005031.

170. Minozzi S, Amato L, Vecchi S, Davoli M, Kirchmayer U and Verster A (2006). Oral naltrexone maintenance treatment for opioid dependence. *Cochrane Database Systematic Review.*(1):CD001333.

171. Carroll KM, Ball SA, Nich C, O'Connor PG, Eagan DA, Frankforter TL, Triffleman EG, Shi J and Rounsaville BJ (2001). Targeting behavioral therapies to enhance naltrexone treatment of opioid dependence: efficacy of contingency management and significant other involvement. *Archives of General Psychiatry.* 58(8):755-761.

172. Tucker T, Ritter A, Maher C and Jackson H (2004). A randomized control trial of group counseling in a naltrexone treatment program. *Journal of Substance Abuse Treatment.* 27(4):277-288.

173. Fals-Stewart W and O'Farrell TJ (2003). Behavioral family counseling and naltrexone for male opioid-dependent patients. *Journal of Consulting and Clinical Psychology.* 71(3):432-442.

174. Magura S, Blankertz L, Madison EM, Friedman E and Gomez A (2007). An innovative job placement model for unemployed methadone patients: a randomized clinical trial. *Substance Use and Misuse.* 42(5):811-828.

175. Silverman K, Svikis D, Robles E, Stitzer ML and Bigelow GE (2001). A reinforcement-based therapeutic workplace for the treatment of drug abuse: six-month abstinence outcomes. *Experimental Clinical Psychopharmacology.* 9(1):14-23.

176. Platt JJ and Metzger D (1985). The role of employment in the rehabilitation of heroin addicts. *NIDA Research Monograph.* 58:111-121.

177. Katz A (1986). Fellowship, Helping and Healing: The Re-Emergence of Self-Help Groups. *Nonprofit and Voluntary Sector Quarterly.* 15(2):4-13.

178. van Dorp EL, Yassen A and Dahan A (2007). Naloxone treatment in opioid addiction: the risks and benefits. *Expert Opinion in Drug Safety.* 6(2):125-132.

179. Robins LN (1984). The natural history of adolescent drug use. *American Journal of Public Health.* 74(7):656-657.

180. Bruner AB and Fishman M (1998). Adolescents and illicit drug use. *Jama*. 280(7):597-598.

181. Marsch LA, Bickel WK, Badger GJ, Stothart ME, Quesnel KJ, Stanger C and Brooklyn J (2005). Comparison of pharmacological treatments for opioid-dependent adolescents: a randomized controlled trial. *Archives of General Psychiatry*. 62(10):1157-1164.

182. Sells SB and Simpson DD (1979). On the effectiveness of treatment for drug abuse: evidence from the DARP research programme in the United States. *Bulletin on Narcotics*. 31(1):1-11.

183. Nelson-Zlupko L, Dore MM, Kauffman E and Kaltenbach K (1996). Women in recovery : Their perceptions of treatment effectiveness. *Journal of Substance Abuse Treatment*, 13(1):51-59.

184. Ahmadi J and Bahrami N (2002). Buprenorphine treatment of opium-dependent outpatients seeking treatment in Iran. *Journal of Substance Abuse Treatment*. 23(4):415-417.

185. Ahmadi J, Babaee-Beigi M, Alishahi M, Maany I and Hidari T (2004). Twelve-month maintenance treatment of opium-dependent patients. *Journal of Substance Abuse Treatment*. 26(1):363-366.

186. Cicero TJ, Inciardi JA and Munoz A (2005). Trends in abuse of Oxycontin and other opioid analgesics in the United States: 2002-2004. *J Pain*. 6(10):662-672.

187. Chang G, Chen L and Mao J (2007). Opioid tolerance and hyperalgesia. *Medical Clinics of North America*. 91(2):199-211.

188. Gunne LM and Gronbladh L (1981). The Swedish methadone maintenance program: a controlled study. *Drug and Alcohol Dependence*. 7(3):249-256.

189. Yancovitz S (1991). A randomised trial of an interim methadone maintenance clinic. *American Journal of Public Health*. 81:1185-1191.

190. Appel PW, Joseph H and Richman BL (2000). Causes and rates of death among methadone maintenance patients before and after the onset of the HIV/AIDS epidemic. *Mt Sinai Journal of Medicine*. 67(5-6):444-451.

191. Brugal MT, Domingo-Salvany A, Puig R, Barrio G, Garcia de Olalla P and de la Fuente L (2005). Evaluating the impact of methadone maintenance programmes on mortality due to overdose and aids in a cohort of heroin users in Spain. *Addiction*. 100(7):981-989.

192. Caplehorn JR, Dalton MS, Cluff MC and Petrenas AM (1994). Retention in methadone maintenance and heroin addicts' risk of death. *Addiction*. 89(2):203-209.

193. Davoli M, Bargagli AM, Perucci CA, Schifano P, Belleudi V, Hickman M, Salamina G, Diecidue R, Vigna-Tagliati F and Faggiano F (2007). Risk of fatal overdose during and after specialist drug treatment: the VEdeTTE study, a national multi-site prospective cohort study. *Addiction*. 102(12):1954-1959.

194. Fugelstad A, Agren G and Romelsjo A (1998). Changes in mortality, arrests, and hospitalizations in nonvoluntarily treated heroin addicts in relation to methadone treatment. *Substance Use and Misuse*. 33(14):2803-2817.

195. Buster MC, van Brussel GH and van den Brink W (2002). An increase in overdose mortality during the first 2 weeks after entering or re-entering methadone treatment in Amsterdam. *Addiction*. 97(8):993-1001.

196. van Ameijden EJ, Langendam MW and Coutinho RA (1999). Dose-effect relationship between overdose mortality and prescribed methadone dosage in low-threshold maintenance programs. *Addictive Behaviors*. 24(4):559-563.

197. Bargagli A, Davoli M, Minozzi S, Vecchi S and Perucci C (2007). *A Systematic Review of Observational Studies on Treatment of Opioid Dependence*. Geneva, Switzerland, background document prepared for 3rd meeting of Technical Development Group (TDG) for the WHO Guidelines for Psychosocially Assisted Pharmacotherapy of Opiod Dependence, 17-21 September. http://www.who.int/substance_abuse/activities/observational_studies_treatment.pdf (Accessed 09 July 2008).

198. Metzger DS, Woody GE, McLellan AT, O'Brien CP, Druley P, Navaline H, DePhilippis D, Stolley P and Abrutyn E (1993). Human immunodeficiency virus seroconversion among intravenous drug users in- and out-of-treatment: an 18-month prospective follow-up. *Journal of the Acquired Immunodeficiency Syndrome*. 6(9):1049-1056.

199. Dolan KA, Shearer J, MacDonald M, Mattick RP, Hall W and Wodak AD (2003). A randomised controlled trial of methadone maintenance treatment versus wait list control in an Australian prison system. *Drug and Alcohol Dependence*. 72(1):59-65.

200. Stark K, Muller R, Bienzle U and Guggenmoos-Holzmann I (1996). Methadone maintenance treatment and HIV risk-taking behaviour among injecting drug users in Berlin. *Journal of Epidemiology and Community Health*. 50(5):534-537.

201. Thiede H, Hagan H and Murrill CS (2000). Methadone treatment and HIV and hepatitis B and C risk reduction among injectors in the Seattle area. *Journal of Urban Health.* 77(3):331-345.

202. Moss AR, Vranizan K, Gorter R, Bacchetti P, Watters J and Osmond D (1994). HIV seroconversion in intravenous drug users in San Francisco, 1985-1990. *Aids*, 8(2):223-231.

203. Gowing L, Farrell M, Bornemann R and Ali R (2004). Substitution treatment of injecting opioid users for prevention of HIV infection. *Cochrane Database Systematic Review.*(4).

204. Ahmadi J (2003). Methadone versus buprenorphine maintenance for the treatment of heroin-dependent outpatients. *Journal of Substance Abuse Treatment.* 24(3):217-220.

205. Johnson RE, Chutuape MA, Strain EC, Walsh SL, Stitzer ML and Bigelow GE (2000). A comparison of levomethadyl acetate, buprenorphine, and methadone for opioid dependence. *New England Journal of Medicine.* 343(18):1290-1297.

206. Kristensen O, Espegren O, Asland R, Jakobsen E, Lie O and Seiler S (2005). [Buprenorphine and methadone to opiate addicts--a randomized trial]. *Tidsskrift for den Norske lægeforening.* 125(2):148-151.

207. Mattick, R. P., Ali, R., White, J. M., O'Brien, S., Wolk, S., & Danz, C. (2003). Buprenorphine versus methadone maintenance therapy: a randomized double-blind trial with 405 opioid-dependent patients. *Addiction*, 98(4), 441-452.

208. Strain EC, Stitzer ML, Liebson IA and Bigelow GE (1994). Comparison of buprenorphine and methadone in the treatment of opioid dependence. *American Journal of Psychiatry.* 151(7):1025-1030.

209. Strain EC, Stitzer ML, Liebson IA and Bigelow GE (1994). Buprenorphine versus methadone in the treatment of opioid-dependent cocaine users. *Psychopharmacology (Berl).* 116(4):401-406.

210. Fischer G, Jagsch R, Eder H, Gombas W, Etzersdorfer P, Schmidl-Mohl K, Schatten C, Weninger M and Aschauer HN (1999). Comparison of methadone and slow-release morphine maintenance in pregnant addicts. *Addiction.* 94(2):231-239.

211. Ling W, Charuvastra C, Kaim SC and Klett CJ (1976). Methadyl acetate and methadone as maintenance treatments for heroin addicts. A veterans administration cooperative study. *Archives of General Psychiatry.* 33(6):709-720.

212. Preston KL, Umbricht A and Epstein DH (2000). Methadone dose increase and abstinence reinforcement for treatment of continued heroin use during methadone maintenance. *Archives of General Psychiatry.* 57(4):395-404.

213. Goldstein A and Judson BA (1973). Proceedings: Efficacy and side effects of three widely different methadone doses. *Proceedings of the National Conference on Methadone Treatment.* 1:21-44.

214. Strain EC, Bigelow GE, Liebson IA and Stitzer ML (1999). Moderate- vs high-dose methadone in the treatment of opioid dependence: a randomized trial. *Jama.* 281(11):1000-1005.

215. Bearn J, Gossop M and Strang J (1996). Randomised double-blind comparison of lofexidine and methadone in the in-patient treatment of opiate withdrawal. *Drug and Alcohol Dependence.* 43(1-2):87-91.

216. Howells C, Allen S, Gupta J, Stillwell G, Marsden J and Farrell M (2002). Prison based detoxification for opioid dependence: a randomised double blind controlled trial of lofexidine and methadone. *Drug and Alcohol Dependence.* 67(2):169-176.

217. Kleber HD, Riordan CE, Rounsaville B, Kosten T, Charney D, Gaspari J, Hogan I and O'Connor C (1985). Clonidine in outpatient detoxification from methadone maintenance. *Archives of General Psychiatry.* 42(4):391-394.

218. San L, Cami J, Peri JM, Mata R and Porta M (1990). Efficacy of clonidine, guanfacine and methadone in the rapid detoxification of heroin addicts: a controlled clinical trial. *British Journal of Addiction.* 85(1):141-147.

219. San L, Fernandez T, Cami J and Gossop M (1994). Efficacy of methadone versus methadone and guanfacine in the detoxification of heroin-addicted patients. *Journal of Substance Abuse Treatment.* 11(5):463-469.

220. Umbricht A, Hoover DR, Tucker MJ, Leslie JM, Chaisson RE and Preston KL (2003). Opioid detoxification with buprenorphine, clonidine, or methadone in hospitalized heroin-dependent patients with HIV infection. *Drug and Alcohol Dependence.* 69(3):263-272.

221. Washton AM and Resnick RB (1981). Clonidine vs. methadone for opiate detoxification: double-blind outpatient trials. *NIDA Research Monograph.* 34:89-94.

222. Gowing L, Farrell M, Ali R and White J (2004). Alpha2 adrenergic agonists for the management of opioid withdrawal. *Cochrane Database Systematic Review.*(4):CD002024. ASHP.

223. Seifert J, Metzner C, Paetzold W, Borsutzky M, Passie T, Rollnik J, Wiese B, Emrich HM and Schneider U (2002). Detoxification of opiate addicts with multiple drug abuse: a comparison of buprenorphine vs. methadone. *Pharmacopsychiatry*, 35(5):159-164.

224. Amato L, Davoli M, Ferri M and Ali R (2004). Methadone at tapered doses for the management of opioid withdrawal. *Cochrane Database Systematic Review.*(4):CD003409.

225. Cheskin LJ, Fudala PJ and Johnson RE (1994). A controlled comparison of buprenorphine and clonidine for acute detoxification from opioids. *Drug and Alcohol Dependence.* 36(2):115-121.

226. Ling W, Amass L, Shoptaw S, Annon JJ, Hillhouse M, Babcock D, Brigham G, Harrer J, Reid M, Muir J, Buchan B, Orr D, Woody G, Krejci J and Ziedonis D (2005). A multi-center randomized trial of buprenorphine-naloxone versus clonidine for opioid detoxification: findings from the National Institute on Drug Abuse Clinical Trials Network. *Addiction.* 100(8):1090-1100.

227. Nigam AK, Ray R and Tripathi BM (1993). Buprenorphine in opiate withdrawal: a comparison with clonidine. *Journal of Substance Abuse Treatment.* 10(4):391-394.

228. Fingerhood MI, Thompson MR and Jasinski DR (2001). A Comparison of Clonidine and Buprenorphine in the Outpatient Treatment of Opiate Withdrawal. *Substance Abuse.* 22(3):193-199.

229. Janiri L, Mannelli P, Persico AM, Serretti A and Tempesta E (1994). Opiate detoxification of methadone maintenance patients using lefetamine, clonidine and buprenorphine. *Drug and Alcohol Dependence.* 36(2):139-145.

230. Lintzeris N, Bell J, Bammer G, Jolley DJ and Rushworth L (2002). A randomized controlled trial of buprenorphine in the management of short-term ambulatory heroin withdrawal. *Addiction.* 97(11):1395-1404.

231. O'Connor PG, Carroll KM, Shi JM, Schottenfeld RS, Kosten TR and Rounsaville BJ (1997). Three methods of opioid detoxification in a primary care setting. A randomized trial. *Annals of Internal Medicine.* 127(7):526-530.

232. Beswick T, Best D, Bearn J, Gossop M, Rees S and Strang J (2003). The effectiveness of combined naloxone/lofexidine in opiate detoxification: results from a double-blind randomized and placebo-controlled trial. *American Journal of Addiction.* 12(4):295-305.

233. Gerra G, Marcato A, Caccavari R, Fontanesi B, Delsignore R, Fertonani G, Avanzini P, Rustichelli P and Passeri M (1995). Clonidine and opiate receptor antagonists in the treatment of heroin addiction. *Journal of Substance Abuse Treatment.* 12(1):35-41.

234. Gerra G, Zaimovic A, Rustichelli P, Fontanesi B, Zambelli U, Timpano M, Bocchi C and Delsignore R (2000). Rapid opiate detoxication in outpatient treatment: relationship with naltrexone compliance. *Journal of Substance Abuse Treatment.* 18(2):185-191.

235. Bearn J, Bennett J, Martin T, Gossop M and Strang J (2001). The impact of naloxone/lofexidine combination treatment on the opiate withdrawal syndrome. *Addiction Biology.* 6(2):147-156.

236. Buntwal N, Bearn J, Gossop M and Strang J (2000). Naltrexone and lofexidine combination treatment compared with conventional lofexidine treatment for in-patient opiate detoxification. *Drug and Alcohol Dependence.* 59(2):183-188.

237. O'Connor PG, Waugh ME, Carroll KM, Rounsaville BJ, Diagkogiannis IA and Schottenfeld RS (1995). Primary care-based ambulatory opioid detoxification: the results of a clinical trial. *Journal of General Internal Medicine.* 10(5):255-260.

238. Wilson BK, Elms RR and Thomson CP (1975). Outpatient vs hospital methadone detoxification: an experimental comparison. *International Journal of Addiction.* 10(1):13-21.

239. Curran S and Savage C (1976). Patient response to naltrexone: issues of acceptance, treatment effects, and frequency of administration. *NIDA Research Monograph.*(9):67-69.

240. Krupitsky EM, Zvartau EE, Masalov DV, Tsoi MV, Burakov AM, Egorova VY, Didenko TY, Romanova TN, Ivanova EB, Bespalov AY, Verbitskaya EV, Neznanov NG, Grinenko AY, O'Brien CP and Woody GE (2004). Naltrexone for heroin dependence treatment in St. Petersburg, Russia. *Journal of Substance Abuse Treatment.* 26(4):285-294.

241. Lerner A, Sigal M, Bacalu A, Shiff R, Burganski I and Gelkopf M (1992). A naltrexone double blind placebo controlled study in Israel. *Israeli Journal of Psychiatry and Related Sciences.* 29(1):36-43.

242. San L, Pomarol G, Peri JM, Olle JM and Cami J (1991). Follow-up after a six-month maintenance period on naltrexone versus placebo in heroin addicts. *British Journal of Addiction.* 86(8):983-990.

243. Shufman EN, Porat S, Witztum E, Gandacu D, Bar-Hamburger R and Ginath Y (1994). The efficacy of naltrexone in preventing reabuse of heroin after detoxification. *Biological Psychiatry.* 35(12):935-945.

244. Guo S, Jiang Z and Wu Y (2001). Efficacy of naltrexone Hydrochloride for preventing relapse among opiate-dependent patients after detoxication. *Hong Kong Journal of Psychiatry.* 11(4):2-8.

245. Cornish JW, Metzger D, Woody GE, Wilson D, McLellan AT, Vandergrift B and O'Brien CP (1997). Naltrexone pharmacotherapy for opioid dependent federal probationers. *Journal of Substance Abuse Treatment.* 14(6):529-534.

246. Rawson RA, Glazer M, Callahan EJ and Liberman RP (1979). Naltrexone and behavior therapy for heroin addiction. *NIDA Research Monograph.*(25):26-43.

247. Abrahms JL (1979). A cognitive-behavioral versus nondirective group treatment program for opioid-addicted persons: an adjunct to methadone maintenance. *International Journal of Addiction.* 14(4):503-511.

248. Khatami M, Woody G, O'Brien C and Mintz J (1982). Biofeedback treatment of narcotic addiction: a double-blind study. *Drug and Alcohol Dependence.* 9(2):111-117.

249. Milby JB, Garrett C, English C, Fritschi O and Clarke C (1978). Take-home methadone: contingency effects on drug-seeking and productivity of narcotic addicts. *Addictive Behaviors.* 3(3-4):215-220.

250. Rounsaville BJ, Glazer W, Wilber CH, Weissman MM and Kleber HD (1983). Short-term interpersonal psychotherapy in methadone-maintained opiate addicts. *Archives of General Psychiatry.* 40(6):629-636.

251. Stitzer ML, Iguchi MY and Felch LJ (1992). Contingent take-home incentive: effects on drug use of methadone maintenance patients. *Journal of Consulting and Clinical Psychology.* 60(6):927-934.

252. Thornton PI, Igleheart HC and Silverman LH (1987). Subliminal stimulation of symbiotic fantasies as an aid in the treatment of drug abusers. *International Journal of Addiction.* 22(8):751-765.

253. Woody GE, McLellan AT, Luborsky L and O'Brien CP (1995). Psychotherapy in community methadone programs: a validation study. *American Journal of Psychiatry.* 152(9):1302-1308.

254. Abbott PJ, Weller SB, Delaney HD and Moore BA (1998). Community reinforcement approach in the treatment of opiate addicts. *American Journal of Drug and Alcohol Abuse.* 24(1):17-30.

255. Iguchi MY, Belding MA, Morral AR, Lamb RJ and Husband SD (1997). Reinforcing operants other than abstinence in drug abuse treatment: an effective alternative for reducing drug use. *Journal of Consulting and Clinical Psychology.* 65(3):421-428.

256. Woody GE, Luborsky L, McLellan AT, O'Brien CP, Beck AT, Blaine J, Herman I and Hole A (1983). Psychotherapy for opiate addicts. Does it help? *Archives of General Psychiatry.* 40(6):639-645.

257. Amato L, Minozzi S, Davoli M, Vecchi S, Ferri M and Mayet S (2004). Psychosocial combined with agonist maintenance treatments versus agonist maintenance treatments alone for treatment of opioid dependence. *Cochrane Database Systematic Review.*(4):CD004147.

258. Bickel WK, Amass L, Higgins ST, Badger GJ and Esch RA (1997). Effects of adding behavioral treatment to opioid detoxification with buprenorphine. *Journal of Consulting and Clinical Psychology.* 65(5):803-810.

259. Higgins ST, Stitzer ML, Bigelow GE and Liebson IA (1984). Contingent methadone dose increases as a method for reducing illicit opiate use in detoxification patients. *NIDA Research Monograph.* 55:178-184.

260. McCaul ME, Stitzer ML, Bigelow GE and Liebson IA (1984). Contingency management interventions: effects on treatment outcome during methadone detoxification. *Journal of Applied Behavioral Analysis.* 17(1):35-43.

261. Rawson RA, Mann AJ, Tennant FS, Jr. and Clabough D (1983). Efficacy of psychotherapeutic counselling during 21-day ambulatory heroin detoxification. *NIDA Research Monograph.* 43:310-314.

262. Robles E, Stitzer ML, Strain EC, Bigelow GE and Silverman K (2002). Voucher-based reinforcement of opiate abstinence during methadone detoxification. *Drug and Alcohol Dependence.* 65(2):179-189.

263. Yandoli D, Eisler I, Robbins C, Mulleady G and Dare C (2002). A comparative study of family therapy in the treatment of opiate users in a London drug clinic. *The Association for Family Therapy and Systemic Practice.* 24(4):402-422.

264. Dawe S, Powell J, Richards D, Gossop M, Marks I, Strang J and Gray JA (1993). Does post-withdrawal cue exposure improve outcome in opiate addiction? A controlled trial. *Addiction.* 88(9):1233-1245.

265. Gruber K, Chutuape MA and Stitzer ML (2000). Reinforcement-based intensive outpatient treatment for inner city opiate abusers: a short-term evaluation. *Drug and Alcohol Dependence.* 57(3):211-223.

266. Katz EC, Chutuape MA, Jones HE and Stitzer ML (2002). Voucher reinforcement for heroin and cocaine abstinence in an outpatient drug-free program. *Experimental Clinical Psychopharmacology.* 10(2):136-143.

267. Chiang CN and Hawks RL (2003). Pharmacokinetics of the combination tablet of buprenorphine and naloxone. *Drug and Alcohol Dependence.* 70(2 Suppl):S39-47.

268. Mendelson J, Jones RT, Fernandez I, Welm S, Melby AK and Baggott MJ (1996). Buprenorphine and naloxone interactions in opiate-dependent volunteers. *Clinical Pharmacology and Therapeutics.* 60(1):105-114.

269. Comer SD, Walker EA and Collins ED (2005). Buprenorphine/naloxone reduces the reinforcing and subjective effects of heroin in heroin-dependent volunteers. *Psychopharmacology (Berl).* 181(4):664-675.

270. Stoller KB, Bigelow GE, Walsh SL and Strain EC (2001). Effects of buprenorphine/naloxone in opioid-dependent humans. *Psychopharmacology (Berl).* 154(3):230-242.

271. Strain EC, Stoller K, Walsh SL and Bigelow GE (2000). Effects of buprenorphine versus buprenorphine/naloxone tablets in non-dependent opioid abusers. *Psychopharmacology (Berl).* 148(4):374-383.

272. Harris DS, Jones RT, Welm S, Upton RA, Lin E and Mendelson J (2000). Buprenorphine and naloxone co-administration in opiate-dependent patients stabilized on sublingual buprenorphine. *Drug and Alcohol Dependence.* 61(1):85-94.

273. Kim S, Wagner HN, Jr., Villemagne VL, Kao PF, Dannals RF, Ravert HT, Joh T, Dixon RB and Civelek AC (1997). Longer occupancy of opioid receptors by nalmefene compared to naloxone as measured in vivo by a dual-detector system. *Journal of Nuclear Medicine.* 38(11):1726-1731.

274. Arizona Center for Education and Research on Therapeutics (2008). *Drugs that Prolong the QT Interval and/or Induce Torsades de Pointes Ventricular Arrhythmia.* http://www.qtdrugs.org/medical-pros/drug-lists/drug-lists.cfm (Accessed 2008 July 16).

275. Eap CB, Buclin T and Baumann P (2002). Interindividual variability of the clinical pharmacokinetics of methadone: implications for the treatment of opioid dependence. *Clinical Pharmacokinetics,* 41(14):1153-1193.

276. Kharasch ED, Hoffer C, Whittington D and Sheffels P (2004). Role of hepatic and intestinal cytochrome P450 3A and 2B6 in the metabolism, disposition, and miotic effects of methadone. *Clinical Pharmacology and Therapeutics.* 76(3):250-269.

277. Lugo RA, Satterfield KL and Kern SE (2005). Pharmacokinetics of methadone. *Journal of Pain and Palliative Care Pharmacotherapy.* 19(4):13-24.

278. Eap CB, Buclin T and Baumann P (2002). Interindividual variability of the clinical pharmacokinetics of methadone: implications for the treatment of opioid dependence. *Clinical Pharmacokinetics.* 41(14):1153-1193.

279. Benmebarek M, Devaud C, Gex-Fabry M, Powell Golay K, Brogli C, Baumann P, Gravier B and Eap CB (2004). Effects of grapefruit juice on the pharmacokinetics of the enantiomers of methadone. *Clinical Pharmacology and Therapeutics.* 76(1):55-63.

280. Crettol S, Deglon JJ, Besson J, Croquette-Krokkar M, Gothuey I, Hammig R, Monnat M, Huttemann H, Baumann P and Eap CB (2005). Methadone enantiomer plasma levels, CYP2B6, CYP2C19, and CYP2C9 genotypes, and response to treatment. *Clinical Pharmacology and Therapeutics.* 78(6):593-604.

281. Crettol S, Deglon JJ, Besson J, Croquette-Krokar M, Hammig R, Gothuey I, Monnat M and Eap CB (2006). ABCB1 and cytochrome P450 genotypes and phenotypes: influence on methadone plasma levels and response to treatment. *Clinical Pharmacology and Therapeutics.* 80(6):668-681.

282. American Society of Health System Pharmacists (2006). *American Hospital Formulary Service Drug Information*

283. Wang JS and DeVane CL (2003). Involvement of CYP3A4, CYP2C8, and CYP2D6 in the metabolism of (R)- and (S)-methadone in vitro. *Drug Metabolism and Disposition.* 31(6):742-747.

284. World Health Organization (in press). *Chronic HIV Care with ARV Therapy and Prevention including IDU_HIV Co-management: Interim Guidelines for*

Health Workers at Health Centre or Clinic at District Hospital Outpatient. Integrated Management of Adolescent and Adult Illness. Geneva, WHO.

285. World Health Organization (2006). *Antiretroviral therapy for HIV infection in adults and adolescents: recommendations for a public health approach - 2006 rev.* Geneva, WHO.

286. Panel on Antiretroviral Guidelines for Adults and Adolescents (2008). *Guidelines for the use of antiretroviral agents in HIV-1-infected adults and adolescents.* http://www.aidsinfo.nih.gov/ContentFiles/AdultandAdolescentGL.pdf

287. Ferri M, Davoli M and Perucci CA (2003). Heroin maintenance for chronic heroin dependents. *Cochrane Database Systematic Review.* (4):CD003410.

288. Broomhead A, Kerr R, Tester W, O'Meara P, Maccarrone C, Bowles R and Hodsman P (1997). Comparison of a once-a-day sustained-release morphine formulation with standard oral morphine treatment for cancer pain.*Journal of Pain Symptom Management.* 14(2):63-73.

289. Gourlay GK, Cherry DA, Onley MM, Tordoff SG, Conn DA, Hood GM and Plummer JL (1997). Pharmacokinetics and pharmacodynamics of twenty-four-hourly Kapanol compared to twelve-hourly MS Contin in the treatment of severe cancer pain. *Pain.* 69(3):295-302.

290. Gourlay GK (1998). Sustained relief of chronic pain. Pharmacokinetics of sustained release morphine. *Clinical Pharmacokinetics.* 35(3):173-190.

291. Mitchell TB, White JM, Somogyi AA and Bochner F (2004). Slow-release oral morphine versus methadone: a crossover comparison of patient outcomes and acceptability as maintenance pharmacotherapies for opioid dependence. *Addiction.* 99(8):940-945.

292. Mitchell TB, White JM, Somogyi AA and Bochner F (2003). Comparative pharmacodynamics and pharmacokinetics of methadone and slow-release oral morphine for maintenance treatment of opioid dependence. *Drug and Alcohol Dependence.* 72(1):85-94.

293. Eder H, Jagsch R, Kraigher D, Primorac A, Ebner N and Fischer G (2005). Comparative study of the effectiveness of slow-release morphine and methadone for opioid maintenance therapy. *Addiction.* 100(8):1101-1109.

294. Clark N, Lintzeris N, Gijsbers A, Whelan G, Dunlop A, Ritter A and Ling W (2002). LAAM maintenance vs methadone maintenance for heroin dependence. *Cochrane Database Systematic Review.*(2):CD002210.

295. Longshore D, Annon J, Anglin MD and Rawson RA (2005). Levo-alpha-acetylmethadol (LAAM) versus methadone: treatment retention and opiate use. *Addiction.* 100(8):1131-1139.

296. Deamer RL, Wilson DR, Clark DS and Prichard JG (2001). Torsades de pointes associated with high dose levomethadyl acetate (ORLAAM). *Journal of Addictive Diseases.* 20(4):7-14.

297. Kang J, Chen XL, Wang H and Rampe D (2003). Interactions of the narcotic l-alpha-acetylmethadol with human cardiac K+ channels. *European Journal of Pharmacology.* 458(1-2):25-29.

298. Cazorla C, Grenier de Cardenal D, Schuhmacher H, Thomas L, Wack A, May T and Rabaud C (2005). [Infectious complications and misuse of high-dose buprenorphine]. *Presse Médicale.* 34(10):719-724.

299. Vidal-Trecan G, Varescon I, Nabet N and Boissonnas A (2003). Intravenous use of prescribed sublingual buprenorphine tablets by drug users receiving maintenance therapy in France. *Drug and Alcohol Dependence.* 69(2):175-181.

300. Obadia Y, Perrin V, Feroni I, Vlahov D and Moatti JP (2001). Injecting misuse of buprenorphine among French drug users. *Addiction.* 96(2):267-272.

301. Lavelle TL, Hammersley R and Forsyth A (1991). The use of buprenorphine and temazepam by drug injectors. *Journal of Addictive Diseases.* 10(3):5-14.

302. Robinson GM, Dukes PD, Robinson BJ, Cooke RR and Mahoney GN (1993). The misuse of buprenorphine and a buprenorphine-naloxone combination in Wellington, New Zealand. *Drug and Alcohol Dependence.* 33(1):81-86.

303. Alho H, Sinclair D, Vuori E and Holopainen A (2007). Abuse liability of buprenorphine-naloxone tablets in untreated IV drug users. *Drug and Alcohol Dependence.* 88(1):75-78.

304. Comer SD and Collins ED (2002). Self-administration of intravenous buprenorphine and the buprenorphine/naloxone combination by recently detoxified heroin abusers. *Journal of Pharmacology and Experimental Therapeutics.* 303(2):695-703.

305. Fudala PJ, Yu E, Macfadden W, Boardman C and Chiang CN (1998). Effects of buprenorphine and naloxone in morphine-stabilized opioid addicts. *Drug and Alcohol Dependence.* 50(1):1-8.

306. Kakko J, Gronbladh L, Svanborg KD, von Wachenfeldt J, Ruck C, Rawlings B, Nilsson LH and Heilig M (2007). A stepped care strategy using

buprenorphine and methadone versus conventional methadone maintenance in heroin dependence: a randomized controlled trial. *American Journal of Psychiatry.* 164(5):797-803.

307. Fiellin DA, Pantalon MV, Chawarski MC, Moore BA, Sullivan LE, O'Connor PG and Schottenfeld RS (2006). Counseling plus buprenorphine-naloxone maintenance therapy for opioid dependence. *New England Journal of Medicine.* 355(4):365-374.

308. Amass L, Kamien JB and Mikulich SK (2001). Thrice-weekly supervised dosing with the combination buprenorphine-naloxone tablet is preferred to daily supervised dosing by opioid-dependent humans. *Drug and Alcohol Dependence.* 61(2):173-181.

309. Amass L, Kamien JB and Mikulich SK (2000). Efficacy of daily and alternate-day dosing regimens with the combination buprenorphine-naloxone tablet. *Drug and Alcohol Dependence.* 58(1-2):143-152.

310. Comer SD, Sullivan MA and Hulse GK (2007). Sustained-release naltrexone: novel treatment for opioid dependence. *Expert opinion on Investigative Drugs.* 16(8):1285-1294.

311. Sullivan MA, Garawi F, Bisaga A, Comer SD, Carpenter K, Raby WN, Anen SJ, Brooks AC, Jiang H, Akerele E and Nunes EV (2007). Management of relapse in naltrexone maintenance for heroin dependence. *Drug and Alcohol Dependence.* 91(2-3):289-92.

312. Sullivan MA, Vosburg SK and Comer SD (2006). Depot naltrexone: antagonism of the reinforcing, subjective, and physiological effects of heroin. *Psychopharmacology (Berl).* 189(1):37-46.

313. Comer SD, Sullivan MA, Yu E, Rothenberg JL, Kleber HD, Kampman K, Dackis C and O'Brien CP (2006). Injectable, sustained-release naltrexone for the treatment of opioid dependence: a randomized, placebo-controlled trial. *Archives of General Psychiatry.* 63(2):210-218.

314. Comer SD, Collins ED, Kleber HD, Nuwayser ES, Kerrigan JH and Fischman MW (2002). Depot naltrexone: long-lasting antagonism of the effects of heroin in humans. *Psychopharmacology (Berl).* 159(4):351-360.

315. Hulse GK, Tait RJ, Comer SD, Sullivan MA, Jacobs IG and Arnold-Reed D (2005). Reducing hospital presentations for opioid overdose in patients treated with sustained release naltrexone implants. *Drug and Alcohol Dependence.* 79(3):351-357.

316. Colquhoun R, Tan DY and Hull S (2005). A comparison of oral and implant naltrexone outcomes at 12 months. *Journal of Opioid Management.* 1(5):249-256.

317. Waal H, Frogopsahl G, Olsen L, Christophersen AS and Morland J (2006). Naltrexone implants – duration, tolerability and clinical usefulness. A pilot study. *European Addiction Research.* 12(3):138-144.

318. Foster J, Brewer C and Steele T (2003). Naltrexone implants can completely prevent early (1-month) relapse after opiate detoxification: a pilot study of two cohorts totalling 101 patients with a note on naltrexone blood levels. *Addiction Biology.* 8(2):211-217.

319. Anton B and Leff P (2006). A novel bivalent morphine/heroin vaccine that prevents relapse to heroin addiction in rodents. *Vaccine.* 24(16):3232-3240.

320. Kosten T and Owens SM (2005). Immunotherapy for the treatment of drug abuse. *Pharmacology and Therapeutics.* 108(1):76-85.

321. United Nations (1961). *Single Convention on Narcotic Drugs 1961,* As amended by the 1972 Protocol amending the Single Convention on Narcotic Drugs, 1961. http://www.incb.org/pdf/e/conv/convention_1961_en.pdf (Accessed 16 July 08).

322. United Nations Office on Drugs and Crime (1971). *The Convention on Psychotropic Substances.* http://www.unodc.org/pdf/convention_1971_en.pdf (Accessed 16 July 08).

323. World Health Organization (1996). *Cancer Pain Relief with a Guide to Opioid Availability.* http://www.painpolicy.wisc.edu/publicat/cprguid.htm (Accessed 14 July 2008).

324. International Narcotics Control Board (1989). *Demand for and supply of opiates for medical and scientific needs.* New York, United Nations.

325. Handelsman L, Cochrane KJ, Aronson MJ, Ness R, Rubinstein KJ and Kanof PD (1987). Two new rating scales for opiate withdrawal. *American Journal of Drug and Alcohol Abuse.* 13(3):293-308.

326. Wesson DR and Ling W (2003). The Clinical Opiate Withdrawal Scale (COWS). *Journal of Psychoactive Drugs.* 35(2):253-259.

327. Finnegan L (1980). *Drug Dependence in Pregnancy.* London, Castle House Publications.

328. Schottenfeld, R. S., Chawarski M.C., Pakes J.R., Pantalon M.V., Carroll K.M., & Kosten T.. (2005). Methadone versus buprenorphine with contingency

management or performance feedback for cocaine and opioid dependence. *Archives of General Psychiatry*, 162(2), 340-9.

329. Johnson, R. E., Jaffe, J. H., & Fudala, P. J. (1992). A controlled trial of buprenorphine treatment for opioid dependence. *Jama*, 267(20), 2750-2755.

330. Ling, W., Wesson, D. R., Charuvastra, C., & Klett, C. J. (1996). A controlled trial comparing buprenorphine and methadone maintenance in opioid dependence. *Archives of General Psychiatry*, 53(5), 401-407.

331. Oliveto, A. H., Feingold, A., Schottenfeld, R., Jatlow, P., & Kosten, T. R. (1999). Desipramine in opioid-dependent cocaine abusers maintained on buprenorphine vs methadone. *Archives of General Psychiatry*, 56(9), 812-820.

332. Pani, P. P., Maremmani, I., Pirastu, R., Tagliamonte, A., & Gessa, G. L. (2000). Buprenorphine: A controlled clinical trial in the treatment of opioid dependence. *Drug and Alcohol Dependence*, 60(1), 39-50.

333. Mattick, R. P., Ali, R., White, J. M., O'Brien, S., Wolk, S., & Danz, C. (2003). Buprenorphine versus methadone maintenance therapy: a randomized double-blind trial with 405 opioid-dependent patients. *Addiction*, 98(4), 441-452.